Psychedelic Horizons

Psychedelic Horizons

— Snow White
— Immune System
— Multistate Mind
— Enlarging Education

THOMAS B. ROBERTS

ia

imprint-academic.com

Published in the UK by Imprint Academic
PO Box 200, Exeter EX5 5YX, UK

Published in the USA by Imprint Academic
Philosophy Documentation Center
PO Box 7147, Charlottesville, VA 22906-7147, USA

ISBN 1 84540 041 0
9781845400415

A CIP catalogue record for this book is available from the
British Library and US Library of Congress

Cover Image:
Summer Sunset, DeKalb County, Illinois.
— photo by the author

Deep reverence for life and ecological awareness are among the most frequent consequences of the psychospiritual transformation that accompanies responsible work with non-ordinary states of consciousness. The same has been true for spiritual emergence of a mystical nature that is based on personal experience. It is my belief that a movement in the direction of a fuller awareness of our unconscious minds will vastly increase our chances of planetary survival.

Stanislav Grof
The Holotropic Mind (p. 221)

Psychedelic Warning Label

(A former student labeled this this way)

From my own experiences and through readings, I have become increasingly respectful of the power of LSD and other psychedelic drugs. Like any powerful thing, they can be destructive or constructive depending on how skillfully they are used. Among other things, they can concentrate your attention on the most vulnerable, most unpleasant parts of your mind. Therefore, psychedelic drugs should be explored only under the guidance of a qualified therapist, one who has extensive psychedelic training. If you need assistance, most mental health professionals, as they are currently mistrained concerning psychedelics, may be of little help; some could even worsen your state. Furthermore, street dosages are of unknown strength and questionable purity. Until the time you can explore your mind using psychedelics of known strength and purity under qualified guidance, within the law, I urge you to limit yourself to studying the literature and working within professional and other organizations for the resumption of legal, scientific, religious, and academic research.

Syllabus 'Foundations of Psychedelic Studies'
Northern Illinois University

Why shouldn't you put LSD
in your friend's coffee?

See Chapter 8 for the answers.

Contents

Dedication

This Is My Song
by Lloyd Stone

This is my song, O God of all the nations,
A song of peace for lands afar and mine:
This is my home, the country where my heart is.
Here are my hopes, my dreams, my holy shrine.

But other hearts in other lands are beating,
With hopes and dreams as true and high as mine.

My country's skies are bluer than the ocean,
And sunlight beams on clover leaf and pine:
But other lands have sunlight, too, and clover,
And skies are everywhere as blue as mine.

O hear my song, O God of all the nations,
A song of peace for their land and for mine.

To be sung to the tune *Finlandia*

Foreword
by Roger Walsh, MD, PhD

What Are The Farther Reaches of Mind?

What are the potentials and possibilities of the human mind? What are its potential capacities of intellect, heights of development, depths of insight, breadth of love, and range of abilities?

There are two answers. The first is: 'We don't know;' the second: 'More than we think.'

Of course these are hardly new ideas. Remarkable psychological and psychosomatic abilities have been described for centuries as, for example, the *vibhutis* (powers) and *siddhis* (abilities) of yoga, the *paramitas* (perfections) and spiritual powers of Buddhism, and the charisms of Catholicism (Murphy 1992). If we ever doubted such possibilities, the last few decades should have opened our minds. Wherever we look — whether at cross cultural studies, developmental research, states of consciousness, cognitive capacities, self-transformation, or spiritual experiences — it is clear that we have dramatically underestimated our minds and our selves.

Consider the effects of culture, and the fate of geniuses born into preliterate tribes. What do they grow into and how do they express their genius? Probably they become good hunters and gatherers.

Yet the same people born into a contemporary Western culture would have access to the products of the greatest human minds throughout history, and be able, as Isaac Newton put it, to stand 'on the shoulders of giants.' They could therefore become computer experts, aerospace engineers, psychologists, or physicians, and then create further breakthroughs adding to the richness of our human heritage.

Clearly, culture catalyzes and constrains intellect. More broadly, culture catalyzes and constrains both intellect and consciousness. This is the basis of the social philosophy of solidarism which emphasizes the extent to which we are all dependent on the cumulative contributions and consciousness of others. We are dependent on those who lived before us, interdependent with those who live with us.

But the present may barely hint at the extent of our intellectual possibilities. For if humankind is able to survive the swath of self-created global crises we currently face, what might an ordinary person, let alone a genius be able to do intellectually and professionally a few centuries from now? What astounding (to us) intellectual and technical achievements will be standard parts of high school, let alone university graduate education? If science, technology and culture evolve — along with our wisdom to use them well — will future intellectual skills dwarf ours as much as ours now dwarf our preliterate forebears?

But intellectual skills are clearly only a fraction of our mental capacities. Adult development researchers now recognize several developmental stages beyond what we formerly thought of as the ceiling of human possibilities. Given the right opportunities, people can mature to, for example, post-formal operational thinking, to post-conventional morality, and to a transpersonal sense of identity (Wilber 2000).

Meditative practices can catalyze such development, and foster a variety of mental capacities — perceptual, cognitive, emotional and developmental — formerly unsuspected and untapped by mainstream Western culture. In fact, advanced meditators have now demonstrated eleven mental abilities that Western psychologists formerly dismissed as impossible, abilities ranging from lucidity during sleep to control of the autonomic nervous system (Walsh & Shapiro, in press). How many more abilities await recognition?

Developing the head without the heart can lead to pain and pathology, and our very survival as a species may depend on our capacity to balance intellectual and emotional maturity. Fortunately this is possible, and the world's contemplative traditions concur that emotional maturation can proceed far beyond 'normality.'

This maturation encompasses two complementary processes. The first is reduction of disruptive, destructive emotions such as fear, hatred, and jealousy, and for the Dalai Lama 'the true mark of a meditator is that he has disciplined his mind by freeing it from negative emotions.' (Goleman 2003). The second process is cultivation of beneficial emotions such as joy, love, and compassion, even to the point where they become unconditional, unwavering, and all encompassing. Examples include the all embracing love of Buddhist *metta*, yogic *bhakti* and Christian contemplative *agapé*, as well as the far reaching compassion of Confucian *jen* (Walsh 1999). Such emotional maturity is far beyond anything mainstream Western psychology has assumed possible, but initial research is supportive (Walsh & Shapiro, in press).

People can also sometimes change far more rapidly than we formerly thought possible, and such rapid, enduring, and beneficial self-transformation is now called 'quantum change' (Miller & C'de Baca 2001). Of course, most self-transformation requires long, dedicated work, and all too many people underestimate the difficulty of radical change and thereby suffer from 'false hope syndrome' (Polivy & Herman 2002). But the fact that quantum change can occur suggests that we may be able to identify causative factors and thereby accelerate healing and growth.

Quantum change may reflect a fundamental capacity and drive of mind, which is increasingly looking like a self-organizing, self-optimizing system. Given supportive conditions, the mind tends to be self-healing, self-integrating, self-individuating, self-actualizing, self-transcending, self- awakening and self-liberating.

These innate tendencies for the mind to flower, unfold, and develop its potentials have long been recognized in both East and West, psychology and philosophy. Centuries ago Plato spoke of Eros and Tibetan Buddhism of the self-liberating nature of mind. It is remarkable how often contemporary psychologists rediscover related mental dynamics. Recent recognitions include Kurt Goldstein's 'actualization,' Carl Rogers's 'actualizing tendency,' Carl Jung's 'individuation urge,' Abraham Maslow's 'self-actualization and self-transcendence,' Erick Erickson's 'self-perfectibility,' Piaget's 'equilibration,' Ken Wilber's 'eros,' and Aldous Huxley's '*moksha* drive.' While these tendencies of mind had been repeatedly recognized throughout history, they became unavoidably evident, as Tom Roberts demonstrates, with the catalytic power of psychedelics. Based on his observation of many psychedelic sessions, Stanislav Grof would eventually coin the related term 'holotropism' to describe the mind's tendency to move towards holotropic or transcendent experiences and thereby heal and integrate.

Transcendent experiences point to the dramatic possibilities and farther reaches of human nature sought by contemplative disciplines. Enlightenment, *satori*, salvation, *wu*, *fana*, *moksha*: these are possibilities that lie at the heart and summit of contemplative practice. Though formerly often dismissed as mystical mumbo jumbo, they are now beginning to make psychological sense, and they suggest that we are far more than we think. Abraham Maslow may not have been hyperbolic when he claimed that 'Certainly it seems more and more clear that what we call "normal" in psychology is really a psychopathology of the average, so undramatic and so widely spread that we don't even notice it ordinarily.' (Maslow 1968).

Contemplative practices cultivate specific states of consciousness. Whole arrays of previously unsuspected states of consciousness are potentially available to us, states such as profound relaxation, lucid dreaming, meditative and contemplative states, *satori, samadhi, sahaj,* and many more.

We have also discovered utterly unsuspected methods for inducing altered states. Who could have imagined only a few decades ago, how dramatically mind and consciousness would be altered by novel technologies? Yet now we have synthetic psychedelics, mind-brain machines with their alpha and theta entrainment, resuscitation technology and resultant near-death experiences, and even space travel with its induction of the 'overview effect' which recognizes the unity of humankind and our biosphere (Walsh & Vaughan 1993, White 1987).

And what of the potentials offered by future technologies? Super optimists such as Ray Kurzweil suggest that we are fast approaching 'the singularity,' a time of evolutionary quantum changes and unimaginable biological and mental possibilities. Kurzweil's 'law of accelerating returns' suggests that the ever accelerating achievements of technologies such as GNR (genetics, nanotechnology and robotics) — to which I would add neurobiology and psychopharmacology — could result in human-biology-computer mergers that effectively produce a new species, a species possessing what are, for us mere *homo sapiens,* unimaginable and unrecognizable capacities of intelligence and biology (Kurzweil 2005).

But will our growth in wisdom and maturity be sufficient to match and master our growth in technology? This is an increasingly pressing question. The problems are many, and pessimists such as Bill Joy are not hopeful. His famous paper 'Why the future doesn't need us' warns of the devastating possibilities of technologies running amuck, the very GNR technologies that Kurzweil sees as our omega and salvation (Joy 2000). At the very least, our species and planet are at an evolutionary 'bottleneck' as Harvard biologist E. O. Wilson calls it, 'a period of maximum stress on natural resources and human ingenuity.' (Musser 2005). We have catapulted ourselves into what the Nobel Laureate chemist Paul Crutzen calls the 'anthropocene epoch,' a new phase in earth's history defined by human effects on the planet, in which the next few decades and generations may determine our collective fate.

Big picture thinkers such as Duane Elgin (Elgin 2000) situate our current times and crises within an evolutionary view, and see us at a developmental crossroads. We may well consume, pollute, and war our way into social collapse or even species oblivion. On the other hand, we may be able to navigate our way through our current global crises via a forced collective maturation. To achieve this, however, will require development of our mental capacities and inner world as much as our outer one. The challenge of realizing the possibilities of mind is no longer an academic question but an evolutionary imperative. Clearly we are in a race between consciousness and catastrophe, the outcome remains unsure, and we are all called to contribute.

In *Psychedelic Horizons*, Tom Roberts contributes by focusing on the array of possible states of consciousness, and their far reaching implications for areas as diverse as education, society, the planet — oh yes — and for living wisely and well. He demolishes what he nicely titles the 'singlestate fallacy': the idea that our usual waking state embodies all worthwhile abilities.

And one of the most rapid inducers of dramatic alternate states? The answer, clear and simple, is 'psychedelics.' Of course psychedelics can be misused, a fact Tom Roberts is very careful to state. But as William James concluded over a century ago after his own experiments with nitrous oxide, no psychology or science that ignores such curious chemicals and the states they induce can be complete. Likewise, most social scientists now agree that no society that tries to merely punish them out of existence can hope to succeed. (Duke & Gross 1993) Nor can it hope to understand or make use of the full array of human capacities. Tom Roberts's book points us to these capacities, and to our minds' awesome possibilities.

References

Duke, S. & Gross, A. (1993). *America's longest war: Rethinking our tragic crusade against drugs*. New York: Tarcher/Putnam.

Elgin, D. (2000). *Promise ahead: A vision of hope and action for humanity's future*. New York: William Morrow.

Goleman, D. (2003). *Destructive emotions: A scientific dialogue with the Dalai Lama*. New York: Bantam, p. 26.

Joy, B. (2000). Why the future doesn't need us. *Wired, 8*(4), 238-262.

Kurzweil, R. (2005). *The singularity is near: When humans transcend biology*. New York: Viking Adult.

Maslow, A. (1968). *Toward a psychology of being, 2nd* ed. Princeton: Van Nostrand, p. 16.

Miller, W. & C'de Baca, J. (2001). *Quantum change: When epiphanies and sudden insights transform ordinary lives*. New York: Guilford.

Murphy, M. (1992). *The future of the body: Explorations into the further evolution of human nature*. New York: Tarcher/Putnam.

Musser, G. (2005). The climax of humanity. *Scientific American, 293 (3)*, 44-47, September, p. 44.

Polivy, J. & Herman, C. (2002). If at first you don't succeed: False hopes and self-change. *American Psychologist, 57*, 677-689.

Walsh, R. (1999). *Essential spirituality: The seven central practices*. New York: Wiley.

Walsh, R. & Shapiro, S. The meeting of meditative disciplines and Western psychology: A mutually enriching dialogue. *American Psychologist* (in press).

Walsh, R. & Vaughan, F. (1993). Science, technology, and transcendence. In R. Walsh & F. Vaughan (Eds.), *Paths Beyond Ego: The Transpersonal Vision* (pp. 177-181). New York: Tarcher/Putnam.

White, F. (1987). *The overview effect: Space exploration and human evolution*. Boston: Houghton Mifflin.

Wilber, K. (2000). *The Eye of Spirit, 2nd ed*. In *Collected Works of Ken Wilber, vol. 7*. Boston: Shambhala.

There are those who look at things the way they are,
and ask why … I dream of things that never were,
and ask why not?

Robert F. Kennedy

Chapter 1

Psychedelic Horizons – Beyond Tripping

This is a different kind of book about psychedelics. Rather than describing psychedelic experiences or psychedelics' possible psychotherapeutic uses, it describes four future-oriented ideas – ideas coming over the psychedelic horizon, so to speak. I've selected these four because we neglect them in our thinking about psychedelics – especially drug policy – because they illustrate psychedelics' potential benefits for humanity, and because they are just plain fun to think about.

This isn't a book that describes psychedelic experiences. These can be fun, and Charles Hayes's *Tripping* is a good example of this kind of book. His contributors portray their sensations vividly and their feelings emotionally, and often with such detail that they evoke similar experiences, or memories of similar experiences in their readers. Instead of taking a sensation oriented look at psychedelics, this book takes an intuitive approach, asking: Beyond the immediate experiences, what are psychedelics' long-term implications?

In this book, we'll explore together four underdeveloped psychedelic territories. In Part 1, '*Snow White*:

Grofian Psychocriticism,' we'll look at Stanislav Grof's view of our minds as a way to understand works of art — a kind of psychedelic psychocriticism. Have you noticed all the mushrooms — including the red headed amanitas with their white specks — in this movie before? Have you noticed them in children's books, folk tales, myths, and holiday ornaments? This movie and these things will never be the same to you once you start looking with psychedelic-informed eyes. I hope Chapters 2–4 will help inform your eyes. I hope Chapters 2–4 will help inform your eyes.

In Part 2, we'll explore an intriguing lead that notices similarities among intense psychedelic-occasioned mystical experiences, positive experiences that boost our immune systems, and reports of spontaneous healing. We'll speculate about how exceptional healing may occur in spiritual and sacred contexts. Do psychedelic peak experiences energize our nervous systems and boost our immune systems?

If you are someone who is fascinated by the human mind and if you share with me a sense that we can do much more with our minds than we usually realize, you'll especially enjoy Part 3. Chapter 8 'Bigger, Stronger, Brighter — A New Relationship with our Minds' sees psychedelics as one way of adding new cognitive programs to our thinking skills, and my guess is you'll become excited by seeing psychedelics as just one of many mindbody programs we can add to our mental repertoire. In 'The Multistate Paradigm,' Chapter 9, we'll look at some ideas that extend our minds into new ways of thinking. New *ways*, new cognitive processes — not just new things to think about (but they are included too). We'll consider new ideas, which we can think about using our existing, common thinking processes. More importantly, psychedelics are a clue to novel thinking processes (not just new ideas) which our culture has neglected. Some of these new mental processes come from psychedelics, and others come from other ways of producing mindbody states. Our minds are much bigger and capable of more than we have dreamed of. Psychedelics and the multistate mind paradigm they support can increase our intelligence and boost problem solving, claims Chapter 10, and Chapter 11 says because they improve mind studies and other sciences, psychedelics and their mindbody cousins provide an adaptive advantage that makes us more adaptable and strengthens survival. In what may be outright grandiosity, Chapter 12 will make the pitch that exploring and developing these new mindbody states and their cognitive processes are, as its title says 'The Major Intellectual Opportunity of Our Times.'

Making matters more exciting — and maybe scary too — by combining psychedelics and other mindbody techniques into new recipes which produce new mental programs, we may have stumbled onto a way of systematically inventing new mental processes.

As an educational psychologist, I am naturally interested in the implications of new ideas for systematically developing our minds. In Part 4, we'll apply Part 3's ideas to learning, both school-based and outside of school. Basically, our educational system from preschool to graduate school limits itself to developing our minds only in their ordinary, awake state. As if our ordinary state's education weren't enough to keep teachers and professors busy, what happens when we recognize that other mental skills and other kinds of intelligence reside in other mindbody states?

A new version of a well educated person emerges: A well educated person can select appropriate mindbody states, enter them, and use their abilities for the tasks at hand. The meaning of intelligence changes too. All our current definitions of intelligence are based on using our ordinary, awake state skillfully. If we can use other states to solve problems too — and we can — aren't these additional kinds of intelligence? A widely accepted definition of intelligence is 'mental self-management.' Shouldn't optimal mental self-management include the ability to use our full repertoire of mental abilities, those in other states as well as those our ordinary state? In Chapters 13 and 14, we'll see these and other educational questions go through a multistate metamorphosis.

If you're familiar with my anthology *Psychoactive Sacramentals: Essays on Entheogens and Religion*, you may wonder why I don't have a part on religion in this book. For one thing, *Psych Sacs* partially covered that topic. For another, I am collecting ideas for a single-authored book on entheogenic religion. It will take several years, at least, to gestate the book. My ideas are both too raw and too few to deserve the light of day yet.

An INTP Book

When I set sail on my first LSD voyage of discovery at Lake Tahoe in 1970, I knew there was something interesting here, but I couldn't get clear about what it was. Something was intriguing, fascinating, but what? In the next several years, my additional psychedelic sessions were varied, both informative and puzzling. What could I make of these experiences? Being an intuitive in the Jungian sense, I am more interested in the implications of things than the things themselves. Actually, I'm a scarce type — an INTP — that is, on the *Myers-Briggs Type Indicator* (Myers et al 1998). I'm introverted, intuitive, thinking, and perceptive, and this book is a typical INTP's book. Understanding me will help you understand my book.

I — My introversion leads me to pay attention to what goes on inside people's minds — my own mind and others'. As magnifiers of what is going on in one's mind, psychedelics provide a prime opportunity for someone with the proclivity for exploring minds, and this book reports on some of those findings.

N — As an intuitive I ask about the implications of things, about what might be rather than what is: What do psychedelics tell us about our minds? What impact might they have on any number of fields? All the chapters in this book are about psychedelics' implications.

Looking back on my Lake Tahoe experiences, I realize now that psychedelics' sense of portentousness, as Daniel X. Freedman called it in 1968, is one of the things that intrigued me then and still does. *Portentousness* means a sense that something momentous or marvelous is about to happen. Freedman expressed it this way:

> … one basic dimension of behavior … compellingly revealed in LSD states is 'portentousness' — the capacity of the mind to see more than it can tell, to experience more than it can explicate, to believe in and be impressed with more than it can rationally justify, to experience boundlessness and 'boundaryless' events from the banal to the profound.

Having this cognitive process magnified, having a sense of great implications is psychedelic candy to an intuitive's mind.

T — As a thinking type, I react with thoughts rather than feelings, and I like to play with ideas. Combine this with my intuitive's proclivity to note the implications of things, and you see why I think about psychedelics' implications. For example, suppose someone using psychedelics feels a sense of portentousness or sacredness — common enough experiences — do we dismiss these as merely the result of psychedelics' effects on the brain? If so, should we also dismiss them when people have these feelings during their nonpsychedelic ordinary life? What standard(s) should we use to make this decision? Which person or what group has the right to answer these questions? Taking a sneak preview of Chapter 13's 'Central

Multistate Question,' we can ask: How do portentousness and sacredness vary from one mindstate to another? This book is largely a book of thoughts about psychedelics' portents.

When N and T are combined, a person prefers to take a broad-frame view of things, to see the big picture and the overall plan, to see possibilities for the future. Combine thinking with a sense of portentousness, and psychedelics nourish thinking about the future. *Psychedelic Horizons* presents 4 future-views.

P — I haven't mentioned the 'P' in my INTP yet. This stands for perceptiveness, not in the sense of having insights so much as reacting to the moment, to current perceptions. The perceptiveness preference helps people react spontaneously, desire adventure, push the envelope, and think outside the box. Since I am an NT, this P trait shows up more in my thinking style than in how I live my daily life. Psychedelics certainly take one outside the common thinking box.

People with the P preference enjoy change and find routine stultifying. We are explorers who are ready for new adventures — due to my NTness, mind adventures. So when people tell us that psychedelics cause weird, unexplainable, unexpected, indescribable effects, that's more candy for our P-based novelty seeking. 'Variety is the spice of life,' is one of our mottos. I suppose this characteristic helps me enjoy psychedelic sessions' unpredictability — letting what happens happen. I thank my P quality for recognizing the adventurousness that psychedelics offered and for rising to the challenge of mind adventure.

I suppose each type of person finds psychedelics frightening and fascinating consistent with his or her type. At the same time, psychedelics can help someone get in touch with her or his weaker preferences. For me these are extroversion, sensing, feeling, and judging. When psychedelics took me to these less traveled paths of my mind, I felt I became acquainted with more of myself and had a fuller view of who I am. It depends on what parts of our minds psychedelics magnify at any given moment.

When you combine psychedelics with I, N, T, and P, what kind of book do you get?

INTP → broad-scope thinking about psychedelics' implications for the future in a variety of topics.

In addition to this books' content, my writing style(s) express my INTPness. Sometimes I use an autobiographical, first person 'I' as when I describe the personal fun I've had with these ideas. Sometimes I directly address you, the reader. Some of the chapters include nonpersonal summaries of other people's ideas and scientific research, and others (like this chapters' 'Project') detour into little imaginary asides.

Projects

At the end of most chapters, I point to a project that remains for us and the future to accomplish. I believe each of these will provide wide-ranging benefits for humanity, and these goals are some of the reasons I am so optimistic about psychedelics' possibilities. Again, this is not to ignore their problematic and destructive possibilities if we use them stupidly. (If you didn't read the *Psychedelic Warning Label* near the beginning of this book, now's a good time to read it, and take a look at Chapter 8's reasons not to put psychedelics in your friend's coffee, or any other psychoactive drug, for that matter.) These dangers are fully exploited by politicians who pump up fear of drugs, then offer to save us from these fears by electing them. And the dangers — real though they are — are exaggerated by anti-drug government agencies and law-enforcement groups whose funding depends on frightening people about drugs: the more frightening they can make drugs look, the more their funding increases. Meanwhile, they deny the benefits from learning to use psychedelics carefully and wisely. In this book I try to balance the discussion.

Project: Psychedelic Museum and Library

Since the most of following chapters present (sometimes explicit, sometimes implied) a project for long-term human benefit, what is this chapter's project?

In the last year I've known of two collections of psychedelic books and ephemera that have been broken up, or may soon be broken up, and there are other collections that may be dispersed soon if they can't find a permanent home. I suppose there are thousands of people who have psychedelic artifacts from the times — letters, posters, books, and so forth. In my experience, psychedelic craft work — delicate and bold embroidery, handmade pipes, intricately crafted roach clips, colorful tie-dies, intricate carvings, sensuous stained-glass, and so forth — express a bursting forth of creativity energized by psychedelics. It would be a loss to the worlds of arts, crafts, and social history to have these items tossed out.

> (Related fantasy: in an Antiques Road Show of the future, a doddering, old Keno brother exclaims over the fine workmanship of an intricately inlaid wooden hash pipe made by an anonymous artisan of the Sixties Psychedelic Crafts Movement. He whiffs its bowl to assure authenticity, and appraises it at several thousand dollars.)

As a repository of artifacts, graphic art, ephemera, printed and sound archives, a Psychedelic Museum and Library would play a unique role in preserving cultural information that otherwise would be destroyed or lost. One of its roles would also be making its collections available worldwide by putting them online.

Like the Folger Shakespeare Library in Washington, a Psychedelic Museum and Library would become a center for collecting books and artifacts, promoting research, producing and disseminating information. Like the Folger, a psychedelic museum and library would stretch beyond its immediate name and contribute to the overall cultural understanding of its topic, including social history, politics, biology, and related topics. Since psychedelic exploration is an on-going enterprise, it would continue to expand as psychedelics continue to enrich our cultures and other cultures.

What kinds of activities might the Psychedelic Museum and Library support? It would:

- Preserve and protect cultural artifacts and ephemera of psychedelia that would otherwise be lost,
- Provide databases of scholarly and scientific information which will also link findings among diverse fields,
- Present lectures, symposia, speakers, art and craft shows, movie/video series, conferences, performances, readings, concerts,
- Promote new books, CDs and videos, journals, meetings, and 'other' products and events,
- Publish a newsletter, books, and help support existing publications,
- Produce new directions in psychedelic culture yet to be discovered.

The chapters of this book sample a few of the kinds of collections a Psychedelic Museum and Library might contain. The *Snow White* chapters symbolize a humanities and arts wing. (Pardon me if 'wing' sounds too big. Perhaps 'floor,' 'gallery,' 'room,' or 'collection' might be more realistic, but my experience is that I am often surprised at how much keeps turning up whenever I start exploring one or another psychedelic path.) Psychedelic music would inhabit the humanities wing, as would psychedelic archeology, history, religion, philosophy, popular culture, and, of course, literature. I expect author nights, lecture series, art exhibits, and movie festivals would make this wing popular.

The Emxis chapters (Part 2 in this book) point to the vast biological, medical, and psychotherapeutic uses of psychedelics. Organizing and sponsoring professional research symposia would advance our knowledge of psychedelics' healing uses, pharmacology, botany, and many other topics. This wing would also house information on psychedelics' medical uses and contribute to our understanding of our own mental health and our brains.

A multistate mind wing, would focus on ways — both psychedelic and nonpsychedelic — to explore and develop our minds' ability to achieve and use many mindbody states' cognitive programs. Besides our usual, awake state, how many other cognitive programs are possible? How do our mental abilities vary from one mindbody state to another? This 'Central Multistate Question' from Chapter 12 — 'The Major Intellectual Opportunity of Our Times' — would be one organizing theme for this (probably the largest) wing of the Psychedelic Museum and Library. One task of the multistate wing would be to facilitate the discovery and construction of new mental programs (mindbody states) and explore their basic characteristics and possible uses.

'Enlarging Learning' (Chapter 14) presents a multistate approach to developing our minds' fullest capacities, both those of our ordinary mindbody state and those of other states. This education should not be limited to schools and colleges as they now exist, but would also include churches, civic organizations, self-selected projects, and organizations yet to be invented.

At this point, a Private Industry Wing is the most speculative, and also the most promising. In fact, it might pay for the whole museum and library. Will some future company adapt the idea of community psychiatric centers into 'Community Psychedelic Centers?' At first the idea sounds preposterous, but when we look at the evidence (at least when I do, and I am admittedly biased) I believe this idea points to one of the major business opportunities of the next decades. The human future would benefit from legal, controlled, skillful uses of psychedelics administered by prepared professionals in a safe setting. By providing the safeguards of screening, preparation, 'sitting,' and follow-up, Community Psychedelic Centers might someday enhance psychotherapy, religious questing, creative problem solving, invention, and other benefits of skillful, legal, controlled psychedelic use.

Location: Where is the best location for the Psychedelic Museum and Library? Well, the answer is pretty clear, the Haight Ashbury district of San Francisco. Some of the world's major cities boast districts whose fame for cultural innovation gives them special honor and recognition. Paris has its Left Bank. London its Bloomsbury. Greenwich Village is New York's center of cultural-enriching arts and garden of the ideas. When people mention these districts by name, we recognize the locations. 'The Haight' has reached this plateau of cultural prominence, and deserves to be recognized as such. Vancouver, however, has already taken the lead. This beautiful city already has a psychedelic museum, and Canada's growing logical approach to marijuana suggests a similar approach to controlled psychedelic use.

Choosing the Haight, of course, is provided the Haight's current residents want it there. Since the mid-60s, this area has suffered from attracting many undesirable people who had little regard for the Haight's residents. Because the 1967 media played up the erotic, exaggerated the dramatic, and trumpeted the irresponsible aspects of the Summer of Love, people who were primarily interested in fun, frolic, and freakouts invaded the Haight, overwhelming the long-term residents and serious explorers of the mind's frontiers, innovative social thought, and artistic creativity.

Throughout the world people view the Haight as one of the world's artistic gardens and intellectual incubators. Personally, I hope residents of the Haight Ashbury district will see the museum as honoring their district's lasting contributions — albeit willy-nilly — to the ideas and art that flowered there and seeded smaller, similar 'Haights' in cities across America and throughout the world.

> (Related fantasy: What should be the architectural style of the Psychedelic Museum and Library? Should it be a big, imposing, structure with great Greek columns, a marble façade. Should the pediment be resplendent with statues of Hofmann holding a test tube, Huxley admiring an 'absurd nosegay,' Wasson eyeing a mushroom, a twinkle-eye Ram Dass chuckling, and Leary looking at himself in a mirror? I hope not. It *is* fun to imagine how one might decorate such an august pediment and to think of other paraphernalia to fill in the spaces. Hmmmm, this might make a fun fantasy for a stoned evening.)

On the question of architectural style, what comes to my mind is a row of Victorian, Edwardian, and non- descript houses so lovingly, typical of San Francisco. I imagine the front of the museum and library as looking like a regular city block of houses from the 60s time period. One of the houses would actually be the entrance to the museum, and others part of the façade. By the way, this would give architectural historians an opportunity to put descriptive displays in front of each house, pointing out the architectural lineage and features that each facade exemplifies. People would learn about the psychedelic times even before entering the museum. To add a note of authenticity, a hippie might be panhandling on the sidewalk: 'Spare change? Spare change?' Donations, of course, go the museum's endowment fund.

When entering, instead of the usual visually sterile museum galleries, visitors would enter replicas of recreated rooms from the period, with rock posters, paraphernalia, India prints, and other 60s accoutrements. The front part of the building, at least, would be a whiff of cultural patchouli, a 'living museum' of the times. Docents could wander around pretending to be stoned and grooving on the displays. Whether or not the whole Psychedelic Museum and Library would be in this style is another question. There are problems of keeping the temperature, light, and humidity controlled to preserve the books and artifacts.

I like to think of two other features of the museum and library as an auditorium for professional meetings, and if the funding is sufficient, the museum and library could sponsor research on psychedelics and psychedelia. Other uses of the auditorium include music – both traditional psychedelic and a venue for new bands descended from their psychedelic forbears. To my surprise and delight, there has been a steady flow of videotapes about psychedelics. Authors could celebrate their new books' publication there.

(Related fantasy: of course, the museum's 'Head Shop' would offer guests the usual sorts of things museum shops sell plus exhibit-appropriate goods: prints, books, incense, post cards, replicas, sun-catchers, CDs, T-shirts, etc. How about a bumper sticker?

> **I left my heart in San Francisco.**
> **I left my mind at the Psychedelic Museum and Library.**

The Munchies Cafeteria would feature guerilla cookies, Screaming Yellow Zonkers, brown rice, mu tea, Ho Chi Min Burgers, and similar culinary treats. The employees' lounge wouldn't be smoke-free. It would be smoke-required.)

How could such an educational and cultural institution be funded? A wealthy patron would certainly be best. Other patrons might have a gallery or collection named after them. Perhaps a future company such as the one mentioned above whose service is providing legal, professionally guided psychedelic experiences for carefully screened and prepared patrons will be part of the answer.

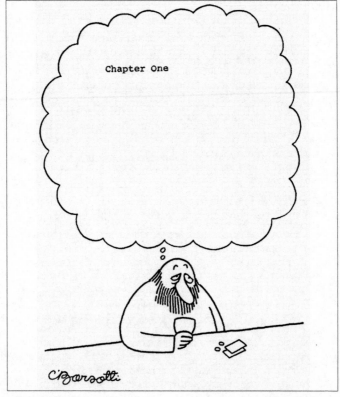

PART ONE

*Snow White:
Grofian Psychocriticism*

The passage of the mythological hero may be over-ground, incidentally; fundamentally it is inward — into depths where obscure resistances are over-come, and long lost forgotten powers are revivified, to be made available for the transfiguration of the world.

Joseph Campbell
The Hero with a Thousand Faces (p. 29)

Chapter 2

Sometimes It's Lucky
to be a Professor

One of the advantages of living in a university community is that the townspeople develop some tolerance for odd behavior — on the part of both students and their professors. Clipboard in hand, I was a beneficiary of this tolerance several years ago when I attended the Saturday matinee, Saturday evening show, and Sunday matinee of Disney's *Snow White and the Seven Dwarfs*. Sitting near the front so that I'd have enough light, I studiously scribbled notes while around me children and their parents divided their attention between the silver-screen adventures of the pubescent heroine and the pragmatic pitfalls of popcorn, gaining the attention of friends from school, spilled soft drinks, and going to the restroom alone and finding one's way back alone.

Seated in niches to the upper left and right of the stage, two gold-painted statues of Rameses II, each 10 feet high, presided over twentieth century versions of the hero legend on the screen and rites of passage to middle childhood in the orchestra.

Built in 1929 in the wake of America's fascination with Egyptiana following the opening of King Tut's tomb seven years earlier, the Egyptian Theatre in DeKalb, Illinois, was not yet a historical landmark. Several toes of one pharaoh revealed that even God-kings may have feet of plaster. Part of a pyramid had sloughed off the right-hand wall, and overhead the formerly twinkling stars of the ancient Egyptian sky had all burned out their bulbs.

It was the weekend following Easter, and I had just returned from a professional annual pilgrimage. As they do each year during the post-Easter week, the Research Department of the Menninger Foundation holds a week-long conference at Council Grove, Kansas, a town named for Indian councils held there in pre-Santa Fe Trail days. 'Council Grove,' as the conference is known familiarly, intentionally publishes no proceedings and discourages coverage by both professional and public press. This is done in order to allow the participants a safe environment in which to try out new ideas and speculations before they are ready to be published or presented at professional meetings. Early research in biofeedback, shamanic healing, meditation, psychedelic drugs, imagery, Eastern philosophies, spiritual psychologies, and similar mindbody topics made their appearance at Council Grove several years before being presented to professional groups and the general public.

As is often the case at professional meetings, the informal get-togethers are as important as the formal presentations. One evening at dinner my companions mentioned that the seven dwarfs in *Snow White* are a fairy tale expression of this often mystical number. They said that in certain parts of Buddhism, Hinduism, Christianity, and in some esoteric Western psychologies the number seven carries special importance. Each dwarf, they said, was a personification of one of the seven chakras in Hinduism. Hence my scribbling attendances at the movie described above.

The Seven Chakras

In Tibetan Buddhism, Hinduism, and some related religions, chakras are understood as centers of psychospiritual development located within the human body. While we Westerners usually consider these belief systems as religions, in reality they are combined religions, philosophies, and psychologies rolled into one. Their views of the human mind are central to all of them. Although there are some variations in the chakra system from one sect to another, there is agreement on most of the basics. From a Western viewpoint, which is more skeptical on spiritual matters, chakras might be considered hypothetical constructs — useful ideas whose material reality is speculative.

Physiologically each chakra is associated with a nexus of nerves, a location along the spine or head, and a gland or glands. Psychologically, each is associated with a value system, personality characteristics, and levels of psychological and spiritual development. Some religious and esoteric systems also associate them with colors, sounds, shapes, jewels, lotus flowers, and so on and on and on. Writings about chakras are elaborate, esoteric, and far beyond the scope of this chapter.

For our purposes it is enough to note that they exist in a very deep part of the human mind or psyche, a level much deeper than most Western psychologists consider. Within these psychologies, the full development of a spiritually and psychologically healthy personality cannot take place unless each chakra is clean, active, and an open conduit for spiritual energy. In *Snow White* we will see our heroine working on this part of her unconscious after she enters the transpersonal level of her mind. Possible connections between the chakras and the dwarfs were the original stimulus for my seeing *Snow White,* but they are not the central thrust of this interpretation.

When I arrived home from Council Grove Friday evening, I discovered by happy synchronicity that Disney's *Snow White and the Seven Dwarfs* had just started at the Egyptian Theatre. With chakras in mind and clipboard in hand, I chose a seat between the two pharaohs.

Synchronicity struck again. The next week my transpersonal education class was assigned *Realms of the Human Unconscious: Observations from LSD Research* by Stanislav Grof. To my surprised delight Grof's model invested Disney's movie with meanings I had not expected. That week we discussed Grof's model in class, then made a graduate-student field trip to see the movie yet again. The Egyptian staff looked surprised to see a large group of adults appear for a midweek showing and then sit in a tight bunch together, intermittently whispering, smiling, and nodding knowingly to each other.

The Heroine's Journey — Joseph Campbell

In *Hero with a Thousand Faces*, Joseph Campbell says that although legends, folk tales, myths, and fairy tales are told as if they were stories of external events, happening to a hero or heroine in the real material world, fundamentally they are psychological stories of inner, intrapsychic events. According to this view, stories which persist over time do so because they carry universal psychological messages that activate the psyches of their readers, hearers, or viewers. Stories which appeal only to personal histories or particular times and places may be popular briefly, but their interest will wane as events in the real world change. Great literature, the world's major religions, folk tales, legends, and other persistent stories strum psychological chords that are deeper than one's personal experiences and more universal than the daily events of historical time and place.

Looked at in this way *Snow White* is much more than a children's story. Stretching across the centuries from a folk

> Some weeks ago I received in the mail from the psychiatrist directing research at the Maryland Psychiatric Research Center, Dr. Stanislav Grof, the manuscript of an impressive work interpreting the results of his practice during the past fourteen years (first in Czechoslovakia and now in this country) of psycholytic therapy; that is to say, the treatment of nervous disorders, both neurotic and psychotic, with the aid of judiciously measured doses of LSD. And I have found so much of my thinking about mythic forms freshly illuminated by the findings reported, that I am going to try in these last pages to render a suggestion of the types and depths of consciousness that Dr. Grof has fathomed in his searching of our inward sea.
>
> Joseph Campbell
> 'Envoy: No More Horizons'
> *Myths to Live By* (p. 266)

tale in an oral tradition through written forms and now a movie, *Snow White* offers a way to study human psychological processes. *Snow White* becomes a general case of psychological crisis and growth which represents common human problems and their resolution. Parts of the psyche are represented by characters in the story, and internal psychological events are described as interactions between these characters. When we look at the Queen, the Peddler-Witch, and Snow White, for example, we are seeing a dramatization of an intrapsychic struggle.

Although the connection between the dwarfs and the chakras initiated my psychocritical interest in Disney's version of *Snow White,* that interest was maintained by the excitement of recognizing other transpersonal elements in the movie: Jungian archetypes, Campbell's concept of the mythic hero's journey, parallels between the standard introduction to fairy tales and the meaning of 'transpersonal,' and, most important, Grof's cartography of the human unconscious. Taken together, these ideas deepen and enrich our understandings of this movie and of other heroes' journeys.

Archetypes — C.G. Jung

According to Jungian psychologists, similar folk tales and myths appear among many cultures because they activate deep layers of the human mind that all people have in common. This layer of the mind is not a product of the experiences each person has during his or her lifetime. It is not a layer of personal memories and personal experiences: it goes beyond the personal; it is transpersonal.

Among the items in this part of our minds are archetypes. These are inborn predispositions to react to our experiences in certain ways. I think of them as similar to empty files that appear when we first turn on a computer. Files, like archetypes, are programmed into us. How we use them and what we store in them comes from our experiences. As we live and experience our worlds, the 'mother' archetype, for example, will contain our experiences, first with our own mother, then with other people's mothers. As we experience more of life, we'll add the roles of mother that our religion, culture, literature, and so forth provide us.

Archetypes may also be processes such as birth or death, roles such as earth-mother or wise old man, natural objects such as mountains or sunsets, or man-made artifacts such as rings and weapons. Stories, tales, legends, myths, stories, parables, and even movies and TV shows which include these items add more material to our archetypal files and provoke unconscious responses in us.

Among the prominent archetypes in Disney's *Snow White* are anima/animus and persona/shadow. The persona is the face we present to the world in order to be socially acceptable. The Queen-Stepmother shows this in her obsessive desire to be the 'fairest one of all.' Her shadow is that aspect of herself that contains the characteristics she most dislikes: ugliness, age, and decrepitude. Like that of most people, her shadow is violent and destructive and remains suppressed for most of the movie, but emerges as the Peddler-Witch.

In order to have a full and vigorous life, a person must tame the shadow's destructive impulses and use them in a constructive way. This process of integrating the persona and shadow is psychotherapeutic, and we watch some of it happening in *Snow White*.

Integrating the archetypes anima and animus is also a necessary step to becoming a fully functioning person. We also see this happen in *Snow White*. The anima is the female side of the male psyche, and the animus is the male side of the female psyche. When these are suppressed rather than expressed, they form part of the shadow. In the Queen we see a suppressed anima coming forth destructively in her domination of the huntsman and her instructions to kill Snow White, who characteristically represents the anima's stereotype — pretty, helpless, and weak. If we are to have a well-balanced person, the Queen, Peddler-Witch, and Snow White must become integrated.

Likewise, the animus is split and unbalanced. The Huntsman-Animus, in spite of his appearance as a muscular outdoorsman, is fearful, weak, and subservient to the Queen. He stands hat-in-hand before her as she sits on her powerful throne. The underdeveloped Prince-Animus needs to be integrated with the Huntsman. The archetype group of persona, shadow, anima, and animus need to orchestrate their characteristics into a harmonious whole.

Introduction = Induction?

Is the 'once-upon-a-time' beginning to many fairy tales and legends actually an induction to a special state of consciousness? Consciousness psychocriticism raises this question and presents some interesting points about it. Among the many meanings of 'transpersonal,' Grof proposes 'experiences involving an expansion or extension of consciousness beyond the usual ego boundaries and beyond the usual limits of time and/or space.' Ego, time, and space are the three limits which are surpassed by transpersonal experiences.

These three elements also appear in the frequent once-upon-a-time introduction to myths, legends, and fairy tales. 'Once upon a time' or its equivalent does not merely point to a specific date in the historical past. It tells us we are actually in a timeless, eternal present. 'Once upon a time' is all time. Likewise, 'in a far-off land' does not designate a specific longitude and latitude. It removes us from the real world to 'The Land of Make-Believe,' as it is sometimes called. Imaginary space-time is created by psychological processes, not the processes of physical reality and not measured by a ticking clock. 'We're not in Kansas anymore, Toto.' These phrases and their counterparts take us to the mythopoetic world where the realities of our ordinary world may or may not take hold.

Grof's third element in transpersonal states is the change in personal identity. During introductions to psychomythic adventures, we are given a hero or heroine to identify with. 'Transpersonal' (beyond the personal) includes going beyond personal identity. It does not mean interpersonal, social, or collective; these refer to groups of interrelated individuals and are at base still rooted in the idea of an individual person, people who have individual identities. 'Transpersonal,' on the other hand, means dropping personal identity or putting it temporarily to the side. During transpersonal states, the boundaries of identity are transcended: personal identity expands to include more than what Alan Watts called 'the skin-encapsulated ego.'

In tales of the hero's journey, we are invited to transfer our identity to the hero or heroine who lives in mytho-poetic space-time. Princes and princesses, common folk, children, orphans, Greek heroes, and various kinds of adventurers all serve this purpose well. After disidenti-fying with our personal selves, we can reidentify with the main character in mythopoetic space-time, who repre-sents part of our unconscious.

When space, time, and identity vary, anything can hap-pen. It is interesting to note the parallel between transpersonal psychology and psychocriticism on the one hand and contemporary physics on the other. In both fields, time, space, and identity (the 'objective' observer) become variables.

Does the introduction of *Snow White* or the beginning of any other legend (whether explicit or not) do more than let us know that the story has begun? Like a hypnotist's 'you are getting sleepy' does 'once-upon-a-time' actually help induce a mythopoetic state of consciousness? It's not hard to imagine our ancestors of several hundred years ago slipping easily into a receptive, free-floating imag-ery-filled state. Tired after a long day full of hours of hard labor, almost certainly malnourished (chemically unbal-anced) by today's standards, then finally eating a meal of questionable nourishment and purity, and perhaps drink-ing beer or wine, our ancestors settle by a fire, stare at the flames, and the story teller intones: 'Once upon a time, a long time ago...' How easy it is to drink the mythopoetic cup!

Today, we stare glassy-eyed at television, have a drink or a toke, put on headphones and 'space out,' at home or in a darkened theater. Relaxation, focused attention, chemi-cal aid, and willing suspension of disbelief (the cognitive functions of our ordinary state of consciousness) — the ingredients change, but the recipe remains unchanged across the centuries.

Chakras, archetypes, the heroine's journey, and mythopoetic induction are transpersonal counterpoints to the Grofian theme. The movie as a whole is a pubescent heroine's journey into her own mind. There she will fight psychological struggles and move toward her own maturity. As Snow White descends into her mind, we'll use Grof's mindmap to chart her journey and to identify the beings, challenges, and steps toward maturity that reside in those layers.

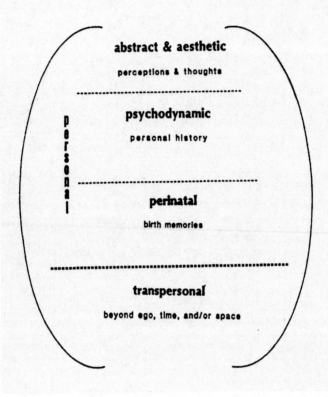

abstract & aesthetic

perceptions & thoughts

----

psychodynamic

personal history

p
e
r
s
o
n
a
l

----

perinatal

birth memories

----

transpersonal

beyond ego, time, and/or space

An Interpretation of Grof's View of the Human Mind

Chapter 3

Snow White – Grof's Landmarks in Disney's Land

As the theater lights dim, we see 'Once upon a time ...' and we know we are slipping into the psychological space-time of mythopoetic reality. The camera's view of a fairy-land castle on a precipitous promontory lets us know we are in a far-off land. What can we expect to encounter during this journey into our inward sea? Stan Grof's work with psychedelic psychotherapy gives a 4-level map to guide us. At each level we wander further into the depths of our mind.

Abstract and Aesthetic Level

When most people think of the word 'psychedelic,' they think only of this level of our minds, the bright colors, sounds, and sensory play that psychedelics bring to mind. In *Snow White* through, we are thinking of psychedelics as ways of plumbing the depths of our minds. Disney's movie, like Grof's theory, pays only moderate attention to this level, but we are introduced to many of the movie's main characters and themes in this level. And we are intro-

duced to parts of our young heroine's personality that
need to be developed and integrated.

The process that accompanies this psychotherapeutic
process begins when the Queen-Persona begins to doubt
the truth of her self-concept. In a classic image of self-
examination that typifies adolescents' self-examination
and concern with what others think of them, she observes
herself in a mirror and asks: 'Am I the fairest one of all?'
Willingness to look at oneself may start just as self-cen-
teredness, but can also be the opening key to understanding oneself and to personal growth. As therapists say,
when a client is willing to examine himself or herself,
psychological growth has started.

Prince Animus shows up astride his big white animus,
appropriately outside the castle walls. Snow White is
washing the castle steps. She is dejected and downcast
while she works; significantly, later we will see her doing
similar work at the dwarfs' cottage with different inner
understanding. In a parallel scene to the persona looking
into the mirror, the pubescent Anima looks down a well, a
classic symbol of looking into the unconscious. As she
gazes at her reflection in the bottom, she sings: 'I'm dreaming that the one I love will find me some day,' and she
spots the Prince-Animus's reflection united with hers in
the perfect circle at the bottom of the well.

This tells us the direction the story of her maturity will
eventually take, but she has lots of personal growth to
achieve first. The various parts of her personality must
mature and strengthen before this unity and anima-animus integration can take place. This first glimpse is overwhelming for her — frightening — so she runs into the
castle, but she is intrigued enough to watch coyly out a
window. The Prince sings a love song, and blows her a
kiss.

Unity Theme

As is appropriate for the love-story aspect of *Snow White,* a motif of love-unity/wholeness-oneness appears from time to time. Since most of our experiences, including images and symbols, are presumed to interact with many levels of our minds simultaneously, they may carry multiple meanings, as does the unity theme. In addition to expressing the Anima-Animus romance and overall psychological integration, this theme takes on additional meanings from the perspective of transpersonal psychocriticism. These are the twin ideas of the healthiest psychological integration and highest spiritual development. To many transpersonal psychotherapists and psychologists optimal mental health and optimal spiritual development are identical. At least they are closely connected and support each other.

When he first appears outside the castle walls, the Prince sings, 'I have only one song, one love.' And his motivation is echoed by Snow White when she sings down the well, 'I'm dreaming of the one I love.' Given the naive adolescence of the characters, they probably do not see the greater psychological and spiritual significance of their quest for wholeness. Although psychological integration forms an overall theme of the movie, it's unlikely that the average movie-goer, child or adult, sees this theme. But motivation and meaning are often obscured. The unity theme is more than a love story; it is also an expression of the desire for the combined goal of psychological wholeness and spiritual oneness.

Dwelling Theme

A minor motif that begins here is the dwelling theme. A house or other building is often taken to represent either oneself or one's life. Although this may not be important in *Snow White,* this minor theme enriches the psychological story. In the Once-Upon-a-Time exposition, the castle is a turreted, fairy tale castle, similar to the castle in Disneyland's Magic Kingdom. As the Prince appears outside its thick walls, the castle appears to be more a medieval defensive fortification. The Snow White (immature anima) part of the personality will forego this fantasy luxury for the humble dwarfs' cottage, while the Shadow-Queen appears later in a dark, foreboding, mist-enshrouded castle at night. Finally, at the very end of the movie, Snow White and the Prince move toward a golden, spiritual castle in the sky, possibly indicating psychological integration and spiritual elevation as well as idealized love.

These introductory scenes also introduce us to birds and animals, which may represent psychic and intuitive abilities. It is common in myths, legends, and children's stories, especially in Disney movies, for animals to have a 'sixth sense' about what to do and not to do, where to go and what to avoid, and so forth. They sometimes act as telepathic agents and clairvoyant messengers symbolizing psychic abilities. We will see this later in *Snow White* too.

By presenting parts of the psyche that need to become integrated during the movie and by starting the psychotherapeutic adventure with the mirror and well, the opening scenes start us on the heroine's journey. As Campbell says, ostensibly the journey is outward into the world, fundamentally it is an inner, psychological journey.

Personal History — The Freudian Level

In Grof's model the second layer is called the recollective, biographical, or personal history level. As the location of both the conscious and unconscious experiences from one's life, it is the focus of most current Western psychotherapies. Most Western schools of psychocriticisms are also biographical schools. They try to explain and understand a work of art in terms of the artist's personal life history.

Memories at the personal history level include both actual events and imagined experiences. Grof's theory departs from standard Freudian psychodynamic theory by postulating that memories are not grouped around complexes and developmental crises but grouped according to emotions and/or physical sensations. For example, memories of guilt, anger, or fear would each form a cluster of associated memories. These clumps, called 'COEXs', are constellations of memories consisting of condensed experiences (and related fantasies) from different life periods of the individual. The memories belonging to a particular COEX system have a similar basic theme or contain similar elements and are associated with a strong emotional charge of the same quality' (Groff 1975, p. 46).

In *Snow White*, the brief Freudian-level scenes can be thought of as either Electral or Laiusian in nature. The Electra complex suggests the daughter's desire for the father (perhaps symbolized here by the Prince) and her resulting fears of the mother, here the Queen. In the Laius complex the father usually shows jealousy for the youth and vigor of the son; in *Snow White* we have a female version of this in the Queen's jealousy for Snow White's beauty and the Prince's attention to her. The Queen then instructs the Huntsman to kill Snow White and bring her heart back in a box.

Perinatal Adventures

The special contributions of Grofian criticism exist in the movie's perinatal and transpersonal sequences. Grof says we unconsciously remember our own birth experiences in the perinatal level. This birth level consists of four 'basic perinatal matrices,' or BPMs as Grof names them. In *Snow White*, the four perinatal stages appear in order for the immature anima heroine during her flight-through-the-woods sequence. Later they partially recur for her Shadow-Witch-Peddler. Each BPM contains certain characteristic emotions, symbols, and themes. Like the COEXs on the personal-history level, the BPMs organize experiences and memories on the perinatal level. We see these themes occur in the same order as birth in *Snow White,* although they may not be so organized during actual psychotherapy.

BPM I – Oceanic Bliss – Sunny Glade

The first BPM takes its overall theme from undisturbed intrauterine existence – 'the Good Womb' as Grof calls it. Imagine all the positive emotions and bodily experiences a fetus might experience in its mother's womb. Everything is comfortable, all wants are taken care of, and the child is floating in a warm nurturing place with no worries. Later in life, BPM-I memories may be warmed-up by real experiences, memories, and fantasies such as happy moments from childhood, vacations in beautiful natural surroundings, and being loved and taken care of by one's parents or others. The feeling is one of peaceful, satisfied, contented rest. After our birth, similar real-life, good-womb experiences are filed in the BPM-I file.

In *Snow White* we see this when the Huntsman takes Snow White to a sunny glade in the woods. He remains at a distance in the background. While there she picks flowers, sings, and finds a fledgling, which she puts back in its nest, She is a fledgling out of her nest too, but doesn't know it yet. In a nice bit of movie-making the camera widens its angle by zooming back, and the sunny glade appears surrounded by a threatening, dark woods.

BPM II – No-exit Hell – Trapped

During birth, BPM II occurs when contractions start and the baby is trapped with no way to escape. The dominant emotional feeling is being trapped with no hope of fighting back or no way of escape. Our later real-life situations that endanger survival and bodily integrity get filed into BPM-II too, experiences such as being locked in a car, trapped in a closet, or other situations that arouse feelings of being caught. It isn't always being physically trapped. Being stuck in a relationship or a bad job produce these feelings as well, and they may recall our own BPM II memories and activate them, both our own birth and our life experiences when we've felt emotionally trapped or cornered. Other common BPM II themes are rejection (which is certainly Snow White's predicament) and unbearable and inescapable situations.

In *Snow White*, this antagonism with the mother during this early birth stage is dramatically activated and symbolized. The vicious-looking huntsman approaches her with a knife. What could be more intense than the threat of having one's heart cut out? Snow White backs up against a boulder as the huntsman bears down on her. With her back against a boulder and with the huge Huntsman bearing down on her with dagger raised, Snow White is in the typical BPM II situation with no apparent escape. Trapped between a rock and a hard place — a perfect expression of BPM II. But the cowardly Huntsman-Animus cannot go through with the murder, and cries to Snow White to run away. She flees into the BPM III forest.

BPM III — Titanic Struggle — Flight Through the Woods
The hopelessness of BPM II becomes the furor of BPM III in Snow White's flight through the woods. During birth, BPM III begins when the birth canal is open and the baby starts moving through it. Unlike the hopeless BPM II feeling of being trapped with nothing one can do about it, there is hope, and the baby can now move and struggle. BPM III is energy-filled. Real-life situations that include effort such as striving, trying to overcome obstacles, working toward goals, and other active, effortful activities draw on the power of our BPM IIIs. And our struggles toward achievements contribute to our BPM III uncon-

scious files, strengthening them. Grof's description of imagery typically associated with BPM II describes the onset of Snow White's run through the woods: '...black and dangerous-looking caverns; treacherous swamps; the beginning of tempests and ocean storms, with increasing atmospheric tension and darkening of the sky...' (*Realms*, p. 144).

Movies and TV shows spend most of their time in BPM III scenes or going back and forth between BPM II and BPM III scenes. 'Struggles, fights, adventurous activities ... intensification of suffering to cosmic dimensions... wild adventures, and dangerous explorations...' (*Realms*, pp. 102–103) — these all express BPM III energy. Snow White's panic-stricken flight through the dark forest has all of these BPM III elements. Disney the artist was often at his psychological best in such scenes. The woods become darker and darker. Clawlike branches grasp Snow White as she flies by. Evil-looking eyes follow her wherever she goes, and loom menacingly before her wherever she turns. Tree branches turn into dangerous talons, and the space around her threatens to close in on her. But unlike the no-escape feelings of BPM II, in BPM III there is hope of struggle or at least flight. In BPM III, the person can at least do something, at least run away, more likely struggle against the foes or toward success.

Another aspect of BPM III is a scatological theme. Urine, feces, mucus, blood, and other repulsive substances occur in symbolic form when this part of the unconscious is engaged. Snow White trips and falls down a large hole into a sewer-like underground river. Tree stumps turn into alligator-like jaws and threaten to crush her, but unlike the situation in BPM II, she is not the helpless trapped victim. She can struggle, and does. The ferocious eyes become larger and more menacing. Finally she trips over a large tree root and falls. The screen goes black.

BPM IV — *Death-Rebirth*

A major theme running through the perinatal level is the death-rebirth theme. Let's look back a minute and follow the death-rebirth theme. In BPM I we saw what seems to be an endless period of satisfaction and unity with the mother. In this infinity of floating life, there seems to be an eternity of bliss and no awareness of death. Then feelings of death enter in BPM II with feelings of being hopelessly trapped in death and decay. Then we move from endless torture of BPM II to the energetic, cosmic, struggle for life in BPM III. Then, Grof says, it is resolved by a death-rebirth experience which becomes the door to BPM IV and a fresh, new day — birth. What is physically experienced by the baby as death is actually birth into a new life.

In the movie we see Snow White give up her struggle and apparently die as the screen goes black. The original 1937 Disney book version of *Snow White,* which coincided with the movie's first release, is more specific about death: 'She stumbled over a big root and fell. There was a roaring in her ears; she still seemed to hear the huntsman crying, 'Go! Go! Go!' But she could go not further. She was so miserable that she didn't care what happened. She wanted to lie there and *die.'*

From Grof's perspective the death-rebirth experience 'represents the termination and resolution of the death-rebirth struggle. Suffering and agony culminate in an experience of total annihilation ... This experience is usually referred to as ego death.' (*Realms,* pp. 138–139)

As during intense psychotherapy, in Grof's theory the death-rebirth experience is both a major crisis and opportunity for psychological growth. It can be the death of a narrower self and the birth of a wider, more mature self. It allows a person to gain a wider perspective on his or her life by ending childish emotional and cognitive attachments, including attachment to one's self. After the death-rebirth experience, the person becomes less egotistical and more dedicated to love and service. Snow White goes through this transformation as she moves into BPM IV.

BPM IV — Dawning of a New Day

The transition from BPM III to BPM IV portrays the crisis and breakdown of a weaker personality organization and its replacement by a stronger organization. To someone going through this process, one's situation in life has changed. We see this in *Snow White*. As she falls into the blackness of ego despair and ego death, the ferocious eyes in the nighttime forest glare at her. After her rebirth a moment later, the same eyes transform into the cute, cuddly eyes of the Disney forest creatures. Squirrels, raccoons, bunnies, and birds replace the monsters of BPM III — rather Snow White sees in a new psychological light. What was terrifying at one minute becomes friendly and inviting the next. As dawn arrives, the claustrophobigenic and threatening forest shapes of the night become the everyday trees of the forest.

In LSD sessions, BPM IV often is expressed in memories, fantasies and images of expansiveness, beautiful colors, sensory enhancement, appreciation of a simple way of life, and natural scenes such as sunrise. Their emotional counterparts are feelings of victory, success, achievement, being born again, and a new life. Several themes appear in the BPM IV sequence of scenes. In addition to the death-rebirth theme, we see that Snow White is somewhat more integrated psychologically although she still has a long way to go. She asks the birds and animals, her psychic and intuitive abilities, where to go, and they direct her to the dwarfs' cottage — appreciation of a humble way of life. For the first time a visual theme appears, one which reappears frequently in the background of the movie from this point on, but one which plays no direct role in the plot.

Shrooms Galore

In the forest glade where Snow White awakens, at the base of trees in the background, are red-capped mushrooms with small white dots on their caps. Thus begins the fungi-festooned-forest-floor leitmotif. From here on in the movie, Amanitas will appear regularly. According to Schultes, world authority on psychoactive plants, the effects of Amanita include: '…a feeling of ease character-ized by happiness, a desire to sing and dance, colored visions… Participants are sometimes overtaken by curi-ous beliefs, such as that experienced by an ancient tribes-man who insisted that he had just been born! Religious fervor often accompanies the inebriation.'

Rumors aside, this is not proof that Disney actually con-sumed Amanitas or other state-of-consciousness-chang-ing plants. Perhaps he chose these beauties for their aesthetic value, just as their popularity in the design of domestic objects and illustrations in children's literature is probably more for their color than their psychoactive properties. Perhaps the appearance of mushrooms, cacti, and morning glories in the opening sequence of *Fantasia* is chance too. Perhaps the Amanita and generic tan mush-rooms in the 1937 cartoon *Mickey's Garden* which appear after Mickey and Pluto are sent into an altered state by insecticide are only chance too. Perhaps Dumbo's flight is merely a cartoonist's flight of imagination. Perhaps other episodes of consciousness-altering plants and drink in Disney's movies are chance too. Perhaps. There are non-drug ways of getting in touch with these parts of one's unconscious, and psychologically aware artists would be expected to perceive and portray their inner voyages via whatever route.

Beyond the Self —
Transpersonal Adventures

Led by her psychic and intuitive abilities, Snow White spots the dwarfs' humble cottage across a small stream. When she crosses this Rubicon, she'll be in Transpersonaland. The cleaning and cooking she does there contains both some unresolved BPM III elements and transpersonal elements.

She sees that the cottage — her psychological self — is a mess, and unlike her previous distaste for cleaning at the castle steps, she now charges right into the dirt and dust with manic activity: 'Whistle while you work.' Working on oneself (cleaning up one's act) is frequently a way difficult psychotherapy is symbolized. As Grof points out, manic activity and wanting to throw a party (the dwarfs' dinner?) is typical of BPM IV if there are still unresolved issues from BPM III. As we will see later in the dungeon sequence, the Persona and Shadow still need to be integrated. At this point little Anima has matured considerably and is taking responsibility for her own actions and goals and is even directing the actions of others, her animal and bird helpers.

In terms of her inner journey we have seen Snow White glance down the well into her unconscious, pass through a brief Freudian stage of conflict with her mother-substitute, move through the entire perinatal sequence, and start her transpersonal development. Now she must go still deeper into her mind. Tired after cleaning the house and preparing dinner, she goes upstairs to put herself into a still deeper state of consciousness, sleep. When she 'awakens' from her 'sleep,' she will discover the seven chakras.

The Seven Chakras

Meanwhile deep within the mind mine, the chakra-dwarfs are busily digging. They aren't mining coal, or iron, or any other metal. They are mining jewels, and in Eastern and esoteric traditions a jewel is located at the center of each chakra. Alternately a jewel is sometimes pictured at the crown chakra at the top of the head, representing a connection between the worldly state of man and matter and the higher state of spirit and enlightenment. Singing 'Heigh-ho, heigh-ho, it's home from work we go,' they march home through the fungi festooned forest floor.

After some cinematic funny business when the dwarfs and Snow White discover each other, they start mutual nurturing and growth. Like a den of Cub Scouts coming in after school, the dwarfs attack the heavily laden table. 'Not until you've washed your faces and hands,' Snow White says. She knows chakras must be clean as well as nourished. In spite of this outrageous request, they comply by washing at the watering trough... all except Grumpy. And there is more cinematic playfulness around the pump while getting Grumpy washed. After dinner the dwarfs teach Snow White a yodel song (mantra?) and dance (mudra?). The following morning the dwarfs heigh-ho off to work, and Snow White picks up her mania for work by baking each of them a pie.

From Persona to Shadow

Meanwhile back at the castle, Queen Persona has decided to do a bit more self-reflecting and finds her rival is alive and living with the dwarfs. Her rage sends her down into the dungeon of her mind, where she concocts two potions. While preparing the first portion, she holds the glass chalice up to a window, and a bolt of lightning strikes it, electronizing the solution. In the language of psychedelia, 'electric' is often used to characterize the most intense psychedelic experiences; for example, Tom Wolfe's book *The Electric Kool-Aid Acid Test*. Disney's *Snow White*, of course, was produced long before the psychedelic Sixties, so Disney's use of this image did not come from this source.

The first portion is a Peddler's disguise, which she drinks, sending her on a prototypical 'bad trip.' She gasps for breath. Her own hand clutches at her throat, and her eyes bulge wide with terror as she is caught in a vortex with no escape — typical BPM II.

Ordinarily, when one thinks of a disguise, such things as changes in clothing, grooming, movement, and voice naturally come to mind. But drinking a disguise? That's an odd idea. Can one change one's appearance by drinking a chemical? Anthropological readings do contain instances of changes in shape and identity resulting from ingesting and inhaling psychoactive substances. Where did Disney get his idea? Was he a student of shamanism? The outward transformation we are seeing is inner, psychological change. The beautiful, young, powerful, haughty vain Queen is expressing everything she wants least to be, an ugly, old, lowly crone. She has become her shadow. The second potion is intended for Snow White. It won't kill her, but will send her into a deep sleep (yet a still deeper mindbody state), which can be ended only by Love's First Kiss.

Meanwhile back in the woods, Snow White has continued on with her manic domestic chores, and her dedication to the service of others indicates she is spiritually more advanced than she was as the simple Anima washing the castle steps. When the Shadow-Peddler appears, Snow White is immediately frightened, and her bird and animal intuitive and psychic abilities try to drive the old hag away. The peddler feigns sickness, and compassionate Snow White brings her into the cottage to recover. In false thankfulness, the Shadow gives Snow White the potion-dipped apple, telling her: 'You will see the one you love.' Personal attachments such as wealth, influence, or power do not tempt Snow White now that she is motivated by transpersonal values, but she still longs for integration with the Animus, for unity and cosmic oneness. She bites the apple, and is off into a still deeper realm of the heroine's inner journey.

Meanwhile back at the mine, the dwarfs are digging their jewels. At least they are trying to, but Snow White's bird and animal familiars are pestering them by pulling at their beards and tugging at their clothes. The dwarfs think the birds and animals have gone batty. Sleepy however, yawns and wonders aloud whether something is the matter with Snow White. They all immediately sense that this is the reason for the birds' and animals' odd behavior, and off they ride on animalback to rescue her, led by Grumpy.

It may be noteworthy that Sleepy recognizes the message of danger and that Grumpy leads the dwarf cavalry to the rescue. Apparently Sleepy was improved by the previous night's cleaning and nourishment for he is more alert now and the one to understand the birds' and animals' frenzy. Sleepy, the sixth link of the chakra system, is located at the 'third eye,' a spot in the lower part of the forehead just above the eyebrows. This center is associated with telepathy, clairvoyance, and other psychic activities, so it is appropriate that Sleepy understands the message of danger at a distance. Sleepy has become more awake.

Grumpy, who is located at the adrenals in the chakra system, represents both anger and excitement — adrenaline — he now is able to focus his aggression appropriately. Doc, who stumbled over his words when he first met Snow White, now also speaks more clearly. Apparently, with Snow White's cleaning and nourishment the chakras are functioning better, although not perfectly.

The dwarfs chase the Peddler-Shadow up a steep cliff, and she is about to lever a huge boulder down on them, when (in good Joseph Campbell fashion) they are rescued from beyond. A bolt of lightning breaks off the ledge where she is standing, and the last we see of the Queen-Peddler-Shadow are two vultures circling. The dwarfs place Snow White in a glass casket in the woods. Together with all her feathered and furry friends, they weep at her apparent death.

Exeunt Omnes

Where are we now in the intrapsychic drama? The Persona and Shadow have been united and obliterated. The Huntsman part of the Animus is forgotten, and Prince Animus is out doing whatever Princes and their horses do in the woods. Little Anima has matured and gown stronger through a series of psychological adventures and now is in such a deep state of consciousness that she appears dead. The intuitive and psychic abilities and the chakras are all quietly mourning.

Suddenly who should arrive, his great white animus in-hand? 'Some day my prince will come.' The antidote for the potion is Love's First Kiss. He kisses her… nothing happens. She just lies there. Is something wrong? Then she stirs and awakens. Animus and Anima are united. To the jubilation of the dwarfs, birds, and animals, they ride off together toward the great spiritual castle in the golden clouds.

Chapter 4

A Thinking Project

Each semester when I teach my *Foundations of Psychedelic Studies* course, the second book we read is Stan Grof's *Realms of the Human Unconscious*. The first is Huxley's *Doors of Perception*. In *Realms*, Grof presents his 4-level view of our minds, including the perinatal level, with its 4 BPMs. This has evolved into one of the class assignments that is most fun for my students and me and is successful in teaching the BPMs. I give my 'Snow White Lecture' (basically, the previous 2 chapters), and in the next class my students use Grof's BPMs to analyze something. We all enjoy these analyses as they present them to the rest of the class. As this is early in the semester, it also helps student know each other and feel at home in the class.

The richness of their selections illustrates how useful and versatile Grof's cartography can be. They analyze movies, TV shows, musical lyrics, daily news events, football games — you name it. I tell them that Stan and Christina Grof acted as special effects consultants for the movie *Brainstorm*, and that starts us wondering whether Hollywood now intentionally uses BPM events to involve their audiences' emotions. Mythic-form movies such as the Star Wars, Lord of the Rings, and Harry Potter series get lots of attention, as do classic cowboy and science fiction movies.

Not all of their presentations are fiction-based. In my memory, one of the most memorable was a woman who discussed BPM elements in the dreams she had during her first pregnancy. Other mothers in my class chimed in with accounts of their first-pregnancy dreams. The BPM themes were powerful and dramatic as only a dream or psychedelic session can be. Another student discussed the BPM elements of taking a shower in the rooming house where she lives and the water often turns cold. Another gave a humorous description of buying a pair of shoes and wearing them to a dance.

Recently a woman from Turkey who took my class wrote such a good BPM-based interpretation of the film *Fight Club* that I encouraged her to submit it to a journal. By the time all the students have given their BPM papers, everyone has learned to spot BPMs in their many disguises. But I like to use Grof's cartography as a door to give my students a wider perspective on thinking and on ideas too.

Kicking it up a psychology notch. In the next class, we start off by discussing additional 'BPM sightings.' After a few minutes of this, I point out how Grof's map of our minds helps us understand things we've known about in a new way and helps us notice things we would have otherwise missed. Because everyone in the class has experienced this, there is general agreement that Grof's 4 layers of our minds and 4 BPMs have enriched our thinking.

Then we step back a bit to see a wider the picture: Think of all the other psychologies and all the ways they might enrich our ways of thinking. There are over 100. We could just as well use their ideas as Grof's BPMs. Some students are not used to thinking about thinking, and shifting gears from the specifics of Grof's theory to looking at it as one of many possible psychological theories gives them a meta-cognitive jolt — thinking about thinking. Often members of our class have run into ideas from Jung, Freud, or women's studies and mention them as additional ways to interpret.

Kicking it up an interdisciplinary notch. I carry on this metacognitive approach. 'Teaching you ideas so that you can think in more ways, is what education is primarily about. One mark of an educated person is the ability to think about things from a large number of perspectives.' Then we discuss the goal of education as increasing thinking ability by giving us more ideas to think with. For some students, this is the first time general education requirements have made any sense to them. 'It's about learning to use ideas from many fields.' The Honors Program where I usually teach *Foundations of Psychedelic Studies* has majors from across the university, so someone points out that there are ideas in other disciplines too. 'Think of all the ideas out there. In fact, people are inventing them regularly. Think of all the ways we've used Grof's BPM ideas. In addition to ideas from other psychologies, we could use ideas from sociology, biology, economics, history, comparative literature, or lots of other areas of study.'

Kicking it up a liberal education notch. And these are just the ideas we're using here and now — in Northern Illinois and at the beginning of the Twenty-first Century. People have had ideas throughout human history, and they'll invent new ones in the future. Like people in other times and other places, we don't want to be stuck with just our local ideas from our times.

Here I digress a bit and ask them: 'In fact, there's a profession whose main activity is inventing new ideas, trying them out, refining them, and passing them along to others. Whose job is inventing ideas and testing them?' Silence usually follows this inscrutable question. Pointing to myself, I say: 'Professors. That's our main job. Professors invent and refine ideas. It's called "research." We also wholesale and retail ideas. In the last couple of days, I've been retailing Grof's ideas to you, and now you can use them to improve your thinking. Your BPM presentations and all the ways we talked about using BPM ideas at the beginning of class show you have learned a set of new ideas and can use them. In the retailing sense I'm like Bob Vila selling you Craftman tools, only I'm giving you idea-tools to think with, not just the latest for the home repair market.'

Kicking it up a metacognitive notch. 'Now here's a bit of a warning. Do you notice how once you start to use an idea, it can sort of take over what you're thinking?' We discuss a bit how they seem to see BPMs everywhere and how in just a week ideas can influence their way of thinking about things. 'Here's the warning. Look out for ideas "taking over" your mind and dominating your thoughts without your realizing it. Ideas are tools to think with, but you should use the tools and know you are using them, not let them dominate you.' At this point I put an overhead on, and we discuss it:

> You do not think about rebelling against something that seems like the natural order of the universe; you do not realize you are controlled by your concepts.
>
> Charles T. Tart
> *Transpersonal Psychologies*

At first reading many of the students think Tart is saying that we automatically adopt the ideas of our times and culture. 'Which words say this?' I ask. It soon becomes apparent that what appeared as a statement about social context isn't exactly what the quotation says. 'Tart's telling us that unless we get some perspective on our ideas and look at them, they'll control us': someone says. A more sophisticated goal of education, we discuss, is to become aware of the ideas we use so that they wont control us, but so we can use them — the tools-to-think-with idea. I see this book to a large extent as a tools-to-think-with book. In it I present some ideas, show some ways to use them, but realize they still need research and development.

So, using Grof's theory as a door to thinking about thinking, we broaden our perspective. Using Grof's cartography to interpret movies, TV shows, or whatever else, we learn and use Grof's theory of our minds. Looking at psychology and other disciplines, we realize it is one of hundreds of ways of thinking. And if we learned them, we'd use them to analyze the things we experience. Then we zoom back again and widen the perspective another notch when realize that all the ideas of our time and our place are just that, limited to the idea-tools we know here and now. Other times and other places have their idea-tools too.

In addition to teaching specific content about psychedelics, I like to use *Foundations of Psychedelic Studies* as a door to open up wider issues about the universe of ideas and the metacognitive view of the wider world of ideas. The course is also a warning not to let unexamined ideas dominate our lives, but we should become aware of the idea-tools we use. Another overhead helps make this point:

> 'The unexamined life is not worth living'
> — Socrates
>
> 'The unexamined thought is not worth thinking'
> — Goggin

I certainly don't claim any originality for these traditional ideas. Good teachers — like Socrates — have been pointing them out for thousands of years. They are the classic fodder of a liberal arts education. Psychedelics in general and Grof's map of our minds are especially useful in making these points to current students.

Because so few students (including those who have taken psychedelics) know much about psychedelics' wider implications for studying our minds, they provide a new easy-to-use fresh set of ideas. The movie interpretations illustrate how some ideas are rich in their implications, and this helps get across the point that there are criteria for judging ideas. Students can begin to think about the qualities ideas have and compare them.

Psychedelic-based ideas are clearly distinct from the clamor of ideas that most students wade through at most universities. Their outsider status of being an 'other' idea is an asset in this way. Having just learned a new set of ideas and used them in psychocriticism, students become conscious that they have done this. And they begin — at least the ones I'm successful with — to think about thinking.

Teaching students to gain perspective on ideas and their own cognitive processes is one of my major academic projects. In addition to learning some specifics about psychedelics' therapeutic uses when we study *Realms*, Grof's maps' richness, freshness, clarity, and distinctiveness leads students forward to a higher perspective on learning as well as a more sophisticated understanding of their own minds.

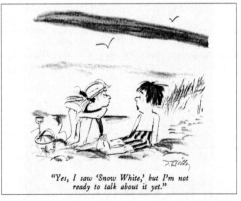

"*Yes, I saw 'Snow White,' but I'm not ready to talk about it yet.*"

PART TWO

The Emxis Speculation

The history of science is rich in the example of the fruitfulness of bringing two sets of techniques, two sets of ideas, developed in separate contexts for the pursuit of truth, in contact with each other.

Robert Oppenheimer

Dear Friend,

Here's another chain letter to copy & send along to others. But this one doesn't promise you a zillion dollars if you send it or threaten you with the dire wolf if you don't. In fact the beneficiaries will be the people you send it to; it may lighten their days & enlighten their minds.

BICYCLE DAY   * * * * * *   APRIL 19th

50th Anniversary

1943 - 1993

Since 1985, some people have observed Bicycle Day on April 19th. This is the anniversary of the day that Albert Hofmann intentionally took LSD in 1943. On the 16th Hofmann accidentally absorbed a bit of LSD, but the 19th was the first intentional experience, when he took what he then considered a minimum effective dose, 250 mics. In <u>LSD, My Problem Child</u> he records that day:

> By now it was already clear to me that LSD had been the cause of the remarkable experience of the previous Friday, for the altered perceptions were of the same type as before, only much more intense. I had to struggle to speak intelligibly. I asked my laboratory assistant, who was informed of the self-experiment, to escort me home. We went by bicycle, no automobile being available because of wartime restrictions on their use. On the way home, my condition began to assume threatening forms. Everything in my field of vision wavered and was distorted as if seen in a curved mirror. I also had the sensation of being unable to move from the spot. Nevertheless, my assistant later told me we had traveled very rapidly.

In this dark hour of ignorance and superstition about psychedelics, you can light a candle of hope and reason. To commemorate the bicycle ride that changed the world forever, let's celebrate Bicycle Day with bicycle trips, sending cards with bicycle pictures on them to friends, joyful picnics, and other festive activities.

Remember Bicycle Day and Keep it Holy

Tom Roberts

A friend and former student made this notice for Bicycle Day™,
and I've used it as the annual announcement ever since.
The original is on pink dayglow paper.

Chapter 5

Binker's Bicycle Day Stoned Idea

The Emxis Hypothesis

Combined observations from biology, medicine, religion, psychology, and psychotherapy point to the possibility of a fascinating relationship among entheogens (psychoactive plants and chemicals used in a religious context), mystical experiences, and the immune system. Entheogen-induced mystical experiences may strengthen the immune system. I call this speculation the 'Emxis hypothesis' — 'Emxis' being a partial acronym of sorts for 'Entheogen-induced **M**ystical **E**xperiences Influence the Immune System.' I built this idea via a two-step process. The first step was on a Bicycle Day, the second from a psychiatrist at Bellevue Hospital in New York.

Binker and I were sitting around getting stoned on a Bicycle Day quite a few years ago. What? You don't know Bicycle Day? Bicycle Day™ is a holiday I invented to celebrate Albert Hofmann's discovery of the psychoactive properties of LSD in 1943. Since 1985, some friends and I have observed Bicycle Day on April 19th. Like so many other inventions and discoveries, LSD's origins stretch over a period of time. In 1938 Dr. Hofmann separated LSD from other chemicals in ergot, a fungus that grows on grains. On Friday, April 16th, 1943, Hofmann accidentally absorbed a bit of LSD and had the first acid trip. The 19th was the first intentional experience, when he took what he then considered a minimum effective dose, 250 micrograms, a.k.a 'mics.' Until that time 250/1,000,000ths of a gram of any chemical was thought to be so small that there would be no discernable effect. But with LSD 250 micrograms is enough to give almost anyone a good solid trip. In *LSD, My Problem Child* he records the 19th:

> By now it was already clear to me that LSD had been the cause of the remarkable experience of the previous Friday, for the altered perceptions were of the same type as before, only much more intense. I had to struggle to speak intelligibly. I asked my laboratory assistant, who was informed of the self-experiment, to escort me home. We went by bicycle, no automobile being available because of wartime restriction on their use. On the way home, my condition began to assume threatening forms. Everything in my field of vision wavered and was distorted as if seen in a curved mirror. I also had the sensation of being unable to move from the spot. Nevertheless, my assistant later told me we had traveled very rapidly (pp. 16–17).

Some friends and I started celebrating Bicycle Day, because of the immense respect we have for Hofmann's discovery and our resulting hopes for LSD's legal rehabilitation and skillful, responsible use in the future. In fact, the primary reason I'm writing this book is to outline some of LSD's possible futures.

Bicycle Day celebrations are making slow but steady progress. The number of Bicycle Day enthusiasts is small, but we are dedicated. One day when I went to a local coffee house 'The House' for breakfast, I was startled to find a CD by a musical group named Bicycle Day. Isaac, one of the House's staff was in the group, and he told me that a philosophy professor at Northern Illinois University (where I also teach) had mentioned Bicycle Day in a class, and the band adopted that name. What a nice surprise! The House is located in DeKalb, IL, but the band eventually moved to Madison, WI. I can't say I blame them.

John Horgan mentions Bicycle Day in his book *Rational Mysticism*, and a quick check for 'Bicycle Day' on google.com leads to other celebrations as well as to non-LSD bicycle rallies and group tours unconnected to Hofmann's discovery.

In our culture, we don't celebrate invention-days, mostly because we don't know the days when, say, moveable type, the waterwheel, or the use of zero were first invented, but I think we should. With more contemporary inventions such as the Wright brothers' first flight, the day the transistor was invented, or when a new medicine was first made or used, we do have records. I think we should commemorate these days just as we celebrate political events — the days wars ended, Presidents' birthdays, Fourth of July, etc. Humanity has benefited from inventions, scientific insights, and medical discoveries as much as we have from wars and politics, maybe more so. And thanks to patents, modern lab records, such books as Hofmann's *LSD, My Problem Child*, we do know the dates of contemporary innovations.

Where does Binker's and my getting stoned on Bicycle Day fit into wondering about the immune system? As we toked, I could feel my hands and feet getting warmer as their capillaries relaxed and expanded. The tension in my shoulders dropped, and I breathed more deeply and easily. A wave of relaxed warmth traveled through my body. A feeling of well-being set in. I rotated my shoulders. I saw Binker stretch his arms and rotate them in large circles, then stretch them deliberately and slowly in all directions.

'Ah! This feels better,' Binker said, rotating his neck.

'Yes, I feel like I've had a tune-up.' I replied.

'Right. I know what your mean.' Binker rotated his
wrists and exhaled smoothly.

'I suppose this is how a car feels when it's had a
tune-up and had all its moving parts lubed and its systems refilled and checked over.'

Like so many other stoned-birthed memories, that one
would have lain dormant and sunk back into my unconscious too. But some time later, I forget how much later, I
received an email from, Dr. Julie Holland, a psychiatrist at
Bellevue Hospital in New York. She was editing a book on
MDMA and asked me to submit a chapter. I suppose she
asked me because I was one of the 4 people Rick Doblin
organized to request the DEA to have hearings on the
medical uses of MDMA. The others were Lester
Grinspoon, Professor at Harvard Medical School, George
Greer, a psychiatrist in private practice who had done a
study of MDMA when it was still legal, and June
Riedlinger, then a professor at Massachusetts College of
Pharmacy.

Dr. Holland asked me to write a chapter on MDMA and
health. Although I started several times, I constantly
became stuck. I really didn't have much to say on that
topic as I am not in a medical profession and had used
MDMA myself only a few times and in both a medical setting and recreationally before it became illegal. As an educational psychologist, my interest was in the mental state
MDMA produced. As you'll see in the next 2 parts of this
book, an analogy I use is to see our mindbody states as
analogous to computer programs, and I was interested in
seeing what program MDMA uploaded and that program's emotional, cognitive, and perceptual areas.

As much as I wanted to be included in Julie's book, try
as I might, I couldn't really think of much to say. As I tried
to write, my thoughts kept turning back to possible links
between that Bicycle Day conversation and the feelings of
health, states of unitive consciousness, and the immune

system. My mind kept returning to an old interest, the link between positive emotional experiences and health, but I couldn't think of much to write about MDMA other than wondering whether the positive emotional experience it often produces boosts the immune system as do other emotionally positive experiences.

I remembered having encouraged a graduate student to look into these connections as part of a study she was doing, and I remembered the additional connections between immune-system and positive mental health she wrote about. I thought of earlier articles in *Brain-Mind Bulletin*, where I first read about how good feelings also strengthened the immune system, particularly increasing the amount of IgA in people's saliva.

In addition to helping digest food, saliva is the immune system's first line of defense against germs taken into our mouths, and saliva is often used as a quick measure of the immune system because sampling it isn't invasive. That is, it doesn't rely on taking a blood sample or lymph sample. A mere swab will do. My writing kept on veering away from MDMA toward salivary IgA and emotionally positive experiences.

It's well known that stress, negative emotions, and life's bad experiences often regulate the immune system downward. I wondered: will our immune systems become stronger with positive experiences? Strongly positive feelings are one of the hallmarks of mystical experiences, or peak experiences. What about the overwhelming powerful experiences that psychedelics and MDMA sometimes produce? Is there any evidence that they might be a booster shot to our immune systems? Would they up-regulate our immune systems? Would they have the opposite effect of negative emotions and stress? I wrote a not-very-good chapter for Julie's book, and sent it to her with some apologies for getting off-target and having little to say directly about MDMA. I wasn't surprised when she thanked me, and said it wasn't appropriate for her book. What could I do with this article/chapter that I spent the better part of a year writing?

Since its beginning (thanks again to *Brain-Mind Bulletin* for alerting me), I had subscribed to *Advances In Mind-Body Health*. *Advances* was started by Eileen Growald, one of the public-spirited Rockefeller cousins. She was its supporting angel for many years. Eventually, the Fetzer Foundation in Kalamazoo, Michigan, took over responsibility for it and is still its home. In 1987 *Advances* published a letter to the editor I wrote. I proposed that we stop thinking about the placebo 'effect' and instead think of a placebo 'ability.' After all, if a placebo is selected because it has no effect, then attributing an effect to something that had no effect wasn't logical. But if the non-effective placebo had no effect, what was causing the 'placebo effect'? It must be something else. Maybe it's a psychophysiological ability that we humans have. It must be a mindbody skill our minds and/or our bodies have, I thought.

So, and most importantly, if we thought in terms of a placebo *ability* rather than a placebo *effect*, we could start to ask questions about how we learn this ability and what goes into this skill. How might we learn to strengthen placeboing? Body imagery seems to be part of placeboing skill, as does having positive emotions.

Is psychedelics' ability to sometimes — sometimes — strengthen our visualization skills a lead to placeboing? Is psychedelics' ability to sometimes — sometimes — produce overwhelmingly positive feelings another clue? Do the similarities between psychedelically enhanced mystical experiences — an overwhelming sense of well-being, ego-transcendence, timelessness, uniting with the universe — offer clues to some instances of spontaneous, unaccountable healing? Do they resemble the feelings in charismatic, religious healing — sacred-energy, resting in the loving hands of God, and a peace that passes understanding? These clues were converging on a fascinating possibility. I had four threads of evidence to weave together — mystical experiences, spontaneous and religious healing, the immune system, and psychedelics — and they were weaving together into one question: Do entheogen-induced mystical experiences boost the immune system?

I made some editorial changes and sent off my manuscript to *Advances*.

Chapter 6

Do Entheogen-induced Mystical Experiences Boost the Immune System?

Psychedelics, Peak Experiences and Wellness

Advances accepted my manuscript, and thanks to the excellent editorial skills of Harris Dienstfrey, *Advances'* editor, the printed version was much improved over the one I originally submitted. It was so much better, in fact, that I asked him to be the co-author, which he graciously declined. My initial response to editors' suggestions is usually to feel angry and insulted at first that they don't appreciate my precious writing. Then, after considering their recommendations, I grudgingly make them (most of them, anyway). Finally, as I look back on my finished writings, I realize they are better, often much better, thanks to the editors' comments. Even after more than 30 years of writing, I still go through this sequence of thoughts and emotions. Maybe some day I'll learn to eagerly open my mail to see how editors' comments can improve my writ-

ing. Harris Dienstfrey certainly improved my Emxis article by putting the pieces together better than I sent them to
him. With some corrections and lots of additions, the
Advances article weaves in an out of this chapter and the
next one. By recasting it into less academic terms, I hope I
haven't distorted Harris's contributions too much.

What are the pieces of information that fit together into
the Emxis speculation? In skeletal form, the Emxis speculation is based on the following 3 observations. (1) The
immune system is boosted by a number of emotionally
positive events in people's daily lives. Binker's and my
Bicycle Day feelings of well-being made us notice that we
felt healthy and that our bodies were functioning at a
higher level physically as well as emotionally. (2) These
positive feelings are weaker forms of similar, overwhelmingly powerful experiences that occur during mystical
states. (3) Under the right psychological state and physical
location — known in the literature as 'set and setting' —
entheogens induce mystical states. Might these powerful
states boost the immune systems just as weaker, non-drug
positive events do, perhaps even more so?

I want to be clear about this. I don't contend that the
Emxis speculation is proven but rather that it offers leads
worth following. There are many unknowns here. In my
own varied entheogenic experiences, powerfully overwhelming states of unitive consciousness occurred about
one-sixth of the time, perhaps less often. Briefer, more
diluted episodes of mystical sacredness occurred over
half the time, but they don't, in my mind at least, qualify as
strong enough to be mystical experiences or peak
experiences.

These mixed results prompt the first of several caveats.
First, the Emxis speculation does not apply to *all* psychedelic usage or to *all* religious uses but only to those occasions when entheogens bring about states characterized
by profound experiences of oneness and the other charac-

teristics of mystical experiences as described in the POTT MUSIC section in the next chapter. Some religions, such as the Rastafarians, use marijuana sacramentally, but so far I know their usage does not produce states of unitive consciousness, and thus falls short of the mystical state that is an essential element of the Emxis speculation. Of course, it would be interesting to know whether less intense strengthening of the immune system occurs under these less intense positive experiences too.

Again, the speculation does not apply to *psycholytic* psychotherapy, which uses small doses of LSD in multiple sessions as a way to help bring otherwise blocked material to consciousness. Since the small doses used as an adjunct to usual psychotherapeutic practices do not produce a mystical experience, psycholytic use is outside the Emxis speculation too.

On the other hand, strong-dose *psychedelic* psychotherapy, in contrast to low-dose psycholytic psychotherapy, uses single, heavy-dose sessions that have the intent of providing powerful psychotherapeutic mystical experiences. In the instances when this experience is reached, the Emxis speculation would look for boosts to the immune system. The fact that psychedelic therapy does not always produce a state of unitive consciousness could be useful in studying the speculation in more detail. Conceivably, if the predominant emotions raised by the therapy were negative as is often the case during psychotherapy sessions, the immune system would not be boosted and might be weakened. And if the patients' stress were unresolved during a psychotherapy session, we wouldn't expect a boost to the immune system either.

By comparing same-dose sessions that didn't provide mystical experiences with sessions that did, medical researchers could test whether it is the drug itself that boosts the immune system or the subjective emotional experience. Both would use the same dose but have oppo-

site emotional tones. Frequently, though, high-dose psychedelic sessions are a mixture of extreme emotions, both
positive and negative.

Psychoneuroimmunology

About the time I thought of the Emxis speculation , I regularly and enthusiastically read *Brain-Mind Bulletin*. When
it arrived at my office mailbox, I'd go to the Junction Res-
taurant, order a cup of tea and read it all the way through.
In those issues, they reported on a new field that linked
people's psychological state, nervous system, and the
immune system. Psychoneuroimmunology (PNI) at last
was finding the biological links between these systems. In
fact, wrote one of the authors whose work was cited in
Brain-Mind Bulletin, it was probably more realistic not to
think of these three systems as separate, but to see them as
one system, our psychoneuroimmunological system. Naturally, I wondered how psychedelic peaks and valleys
affected the immune system. Two standard ways to evaluate the health of immune systems are cortisol and immunoglobulin A. Immunoglobulin A and cortisol? What are
they? Cortisol is a chemical that increases when someone
is under stress and is often used to measure tension,
unpleasant emotions, anxiety, and stress. Immunoglobulin is part of the immune system that fights infections. It's
one measure of how well our immune systems are doing.
Because it appears in saliva (and elsewhere), it is both
quick to sample and non-invasive, making salivary IgA
especially popular with health researchers.

When Binker and I felt especially happy and healthy on
Bicycle Day, were our immune systems healthily producing lots of IgA and very little cortisol? How would these
fluctuate as people went through the emotional ups and
downs of psychedelic sessions? My guess is that the final
emotional state will be most influential in the long term.
But during the sessions the immune system may track the

emotions, closely paralleling its roller-coaster ups and downs.

A cortisol study published in 1998 suggests this. In 'Stressors and Mood Measured on a Momentary Basis Are Associated with Salivary Cortisol Secretion', J. Smyth and his fellow researchers at State University of New York at Stony Brook measured how much stress 120 people felt 6 times a day. Then, allowing time for the subjects' immune systems to catch up with their moods, twenty minutes later they took a sample of saliva. Later they measured it for the stress hormone cortisol. They studied both how much stress each person reported and their emotional mood at the time. As expected, cortisol levels were higher during high-stress times and lower in during low-stress times.

But it wasn't the number of stressful life events alone that increased or decreased cortisol levels. It was the subjects' emotions – positive and negative – that most accounted for their amount of cortisol (stress level). If they had lots of normally stressful things going on in their lives but were in a positive mood, cortisol levels remained low. But if they felt stress and were also in a negative mood, cortisol levels were high. So the emotions accounted for the cortisol levels more than the number of stressful events.

Will the emotional relationship hold true for IgA emotional peaks and troughs during psychedelic sessions? Given the sometimes immense emotional fluctuations that occur, it will be fascinating to know. And if someone has an overwhelmingly strong positive mystical experience, do IgA levels peak too? Do cortisol levels drop correspondingly? If so, we may be on to a clue about extraordinary healing.

This was a really exciting idea to discover. What if we didn't have to wait for extraordinary healing to occur during random positive emotional peaks? Suppose we could produce these peaks — and presumably the healing that accompanies them — in psychedelic sessions? Obviously, not all sessions produced peaks, but there are ways to increase this likelihood. This was the conception of the Emxis speculation. It's gestation and labor? I began to rummage through Northern Illinois University's library, my own book collection, and the Internet to see if I could find links among extraordinary healing, intense emotional peaks, the immune system, and psychedelics. I had wandered away from Julie Holland's request for a chapter on ecstasy (MDMA), but found something much more intriguing.

The immediate place to go was *PubMed*. *PubMed* is the wonderful online research library of the National Institutes of Health. (It used to have a section named *Grateful Med*, but this has been eliminated due, I suppose, to the humorlessness of governmental bureaucrats.) Because *PubMed* is one of the most up-to-date resources on psychedelic research, I include it as a 'Weekly Internet Field Trip' in my *Foundations of Psychedelic Studies* course. I hope my students will continue to use *PubMed* after the course for their questions on health matters. A note for *PubMed* users: Searching for 'hallucinogens' finds many more studies than searching for 'psychedelics.'

I found an amazing amount of research on the relationships between emotions and IgA. (While searching IgA, I was puzzled by the titles of some articles my search was picking up. What did 'Problems in pharmacological evaluation of patients with paroxysmal atrial fibrillation: clinical analysis of more than 100 consecutive patients' and similar articles have to do with IgA? After much puzzling about this and after getting bogged down in their abstracts, I finally realized their author was a medical researcher in Japan, Dr. Iga. Ah! The things you learn doing research!)

During the research, I discovered another reason to be cautious of my Emxis speculation. Even if entheogen-induced mystical experiences do strengthen immune functions, they might not strengthen them enough to influence health. Maybe they strengthen them only marginally. Do positive emotions only help a person return to normal from an emotional low state? Most studies looked only at overcoming negative experiences and emotions, not at enhancing positive ones. In a 1996 study of IgA, medical researcher Arthur A. Stone and colleagues at the State University of New York at Stony Book suggested that the role of positive emotions may be primarily to counter negative ones. Positive emotions may not actually add strength to the immune system above its normal capacity. A year later Drs. H. B. Valdimarsdottir and D. H. Bovbjerg, then at Memorial Sloan-Kettering Cancer Center in New York, looked at another soldier in the immune system, natural killer cell activity. They found that it seemed related to positive moods when overcoming negative moods. This raised the possibility again 'that positive mood may moderate, or buffer, the effects of negative mood on immune function,' as they wrote. That is, positive mood may or may not strengthen natural killer cell activity beyond its normal range.

On the other hand, working with an apparently healthy and non-stressed group of fifth graders at an elementary school in Arkansas, R. B. Lambert and N. K Lambert discovered that concentrations of salivary IgA 'were increased after a humorous presentation.' This raises the possibility that the humor strengthened this immune component beyond its normal range. Perhaps the saying: 'Humor is the best medicine' is true after all. We'll pick up the trail of IgA and how it increases under positive experiences and decreases under negative ones in the next chapter in the section 'The Immune System and Salivary Immunoglobulin A.'

The whole issue of the possible immune effects of peak experiences or mystical experiences is not at all clear because the scientific research has been only within the range of normal, emotionally positive daily events, not the extremes of emotional happiness. Also, most of that research was done in a medical setting where restoring patients to their normal health is the goal, not enhancing health to above normal ranges. The immune effects of exceedingly strong positive emotions have yet to be experimentally studied, but in the next chapter we'll see some non-experimental leads. With its program for researching exceedingly strong positive emotions using psychoactive drugs that sometimes produce mystical experiences, the Emxis speculation provides a rationale for looking at this question and a way to do this research. .

Such cautions and caveats notwithstanding, I think 3 ideas link together. (1) Entheogens sometimes produce mystical experiences, also called 'peak experiences' and 'states of unitive consciousness'. (2) Mystical experiences produce exceedingly powerful positive emotions and thoughts. (3) In daily life-events, lesser instances of these feelings and thoughts strengthen our immune systems. Linked together, these 3 ideas give us two related questions which we'll look at in this chapter and the next. (1) Do the powerful positive affects and cognitions (emotions and thoughts) during mystical experiences strengthen the immune system a great deal? (2) Is it possible to find anecdotal and clinical reports of unusual cures that are associated with mystical experiences and/or the thoughts and feelings that typically accompany them? We can begin tracking these ideas by taking a closer look at entheogens and mystical experiences.

Entheogens and Mystical Experiences

What are entheogens? Because psychedelics select certain emotional and cognitive processes, focus one's attention on them, and magnify our subjective awareness of them, they produce a great variety of effects — sometimes conflicting effects. In this chapter, we are interested in the occasions that psychedelics produce states of unitive consciousness, or mystical experiences. If a sense of sacredness accompanies the emotional peaks, they are called 'entheogens.'

The literature on psychedelics and mystical experiences occurs predominantly in two disciplines, religion and psychotherapy. The word 'entheogen' comes from the religious literature. The term, which literally means 'realizing the divine within' or 'generating the experience of god within,' was coined in 1979 specifically to denote the religious experiences of psychedelic use. The Native American Church's use of peyote as a sacrament is probably the most widely recognized example. Because of the bad press and government propaganda that demonized psychedelics, Carl A.P. Ruck, Jeremy Bigwood, Blaise Staples, R. Gordon Wasson, and Jonathan Ott felt a new and less loaded word was needed.

The classification of a psychedelic as an 'entheogen' comes from its use, not its chemical structure or any other drug taxonomy. The process of labeling a psychedelic as an entheogen is similar to classifying the wine in a religious ceremony as a sacrament, by its use, rather than by its chemical structure or its possible other uses as a food, medicine, or recreational drug.

The scholarly writings on entheogens occur in religion, theology, psychology, archeology, anthropology, sociology, history, law, literature, and a scattering of related fields. With a co-author, I have compiled an online archive of more than 550 books, dissertations, theses, and topical issues of journals that have something significant to say about entheogens in *Psychoactive Sacraments: An Entheogen Chrestomathy*, an online reference/resource. A pile of books on my dresser and two thick file folders in my office await my finishing this book so I can add at least 50 more. Most entries contain from 1 to 4 pages of excerpts. Taken as a whole, but still with widespread disagreement, there is general consensus that, under the right conditions, entheogens may induce experiences that are identical with, or closely resemble, mystical experiences that can be attributed to religious practices such as fasting, prayer, meditation, an ascetic life, or 'the grace of God.'

Religious writings on entheogens contain a large number of complex arguments about whether entheogen-induced mystical experiences are genuine religious experiences and a large number of considerations about how one goes about interpreting these experiences as religious phenomena. My anthology *Psychoactive Sacramentals* and Robert Forte's *Entheogens and the Future of Religion* touch on many of these touchy religious and spiritual issues, and the *Chrestomathy* collects views pro, con, and neutral about the entheogenic uses of psychedelics. The Council on Spiritual Practices publishes of all three.

These sources indicate entheogens do produce mystical experiences, and they resemble intense religious experiences. Internationally renowned philosopher of religion Huston Smith evaluates Bob Forte's anthology as 'the best single inquiry into the religious significance of chemically occasioned mystical experiences that has yet appeared.' With various flavors to their answers, the contributors maintain that entheogens sometimes produce religious experiences.

Since then Huston Smith has written his own book on entheogens. *Cleansing the Doors of Perception: Essays on Entheogens and Religion* is a collection of Huston's lifetime writings on entheogens (with a bit of rewriting, updating and editing). *Cleansing* and *Psych Sacs* (as I call *Psychoactive Sacramentals*) come out of the same series of events, notably a small, invitational conference in 1995 I helped organize for the Council on Spiritual Practices. They happened this way. In 1993 I wrote a manuscript of an unpublished article I titled 'My Entheogenic Religion'. I sent a copy to Sasha (Alexander) and Ann Shulgin. Sasha had just met Bob Jesse who left his job as a vice president at Oracle to organize a non-profit group to focus on entheogens, since named the Council on Spiritual Practices. Sasha asked me if it would be OK with me if he gave my manuscript to Bob. I said 'Sure.'

Bob and I were soon in touch via email and telephone and were considering what steps to take. With the help of some other people, we founded the Council on Spiritual Practices, and when Bob asked me what I thought we ought to do to get the entheogen ball rolling, I gave a usual professor's answer: 'Let's organize a conference.' That was the origin of the Vallombrosa Conference. Vallombrosa is a beautiful Catholic retreat center in an old estate mansion in Menlo Park, California. Other than being about spiritual matters, the conference had nothing directly to do with the Catholic Church and was not sponsored by the church, but Vallombrosa's spiritual atmosphere and its church on the grounds contributed to the conference's spiritual feeling. Appropriately enough, I had known Vallombrosa as the original campus-home of the California Institute for Transpersonal Psychology, where I spent the summer of 1997 on my first sabbatical teaching and learning there. By the time of our conference-retreat, it had moved to other quarters and — reflecting its worldwide scope — dropped the 'California' from its name.

Little psychedelic meetings and conferences are held from time to time, but other than the people who attend supporting each other, there are usually no permanent outcomes. The meetings, pleasant though they are, fade into the past. We wanted the Council on Spiritual Practice's first conference to have a more permanent effect. Another typical professor's solution came to mind; 'We need to publish a book to record the papers and keep the conference alive.' This meant we had to attract people of enough stature so that people would want to read the book. How could we do this? An opportunity arose one day at church.

In 1993 or 1994 I gave a copy of my paper to the co-ministers in my church, the Revs. Bill and Jane Ann Moore, a now-retired husband and wife team. One Sunday Kenneth Smith, then President of the Chicago Theological Seminary, was a guest minister. On the way to lunch afterwards, Bill mentioned my entheogenic interests to Ken in the car, and although I didn't get a chance to talk to him at lunch other than a quick word or two, Ken seemed interested in my take on religion. Later I thought, if we can get an established seminary to co-sponsor the conference-retreat, that might help attract some well-established professionals who might not otherwise come to just another psychedelics meeting.

Huston Smith was known worldwide as a philosopher of religion, and I had met him in 1972 and again in 1975 at conferences in Iceland. These were meetings of what eventually became the International Transpersonal Association, and Huston spoke about his psychedelic experiences and their impact on his understanding of spiritual development. More than 20 years had passed, and war on drugs had pretty well sent interest in the entheogenic path of spiritual development underground. Would a world renowned philosopher of religion be willing to reopen this area of interest? How could I attract him to the conference? Getting the Chicago Theological Seminary to co-sponsor a conference would give the conference some standing other than a bunch of hippies getting together, and that might convince Huston to come.

I called Ken Smith's secretary and made an appointment to see him. I hardly knew Ken, and I had no idea whether he could even want to consider having CTS involved in a controversial religious undertaking; although, I did know that the Congregational Church — now part of the United Church of Christ — had a long history of supporting new ideas and new directions in American religion and liberty. From its founding by the Puritans — originally in England then expatriated in Holland and finally in Plymouth — the Congregational Church was proud of its history of innovation: establishing the public school movement, founding universities, advocating abolition, supporting the *Amistad* survivors, including women in the ministry, and supporting individuals' rights regardless of their sexual orientations.

I would use this historic context as an appeal to President Smith to extend the church's position to be willing to consider and discuss — if not fully support — the possible use of entheogens as an aid on the spiritual quest. I was nervous as I drove to Chicago, and I practiced and repracticed in my head a 20-minute spiel that I hoped would convince Ken to agree to CTS's sponsoring a conference to consider the entheogenic uses of psychedelics without either approving or disapproving this limited spiritual, entheogenic use.

Other than briefly meeting Ken at dinner after church, I had never discussed entheogens with him, and I had no idea how he would take my appeal. He had given me detailed directions on how to park behind his own house a few blocks from the seminary. This was a real help in the heavily parked-up Hyde Park area of Chicago, and as I walked along 58th Street by Frank Lloyd Wright's Robie house on the way from Ken's parking spot to his office, I hoped his kindness was a hint that he would be open-minded to my idea of an entheogen conference and that he wasn't just being gracious by helping an out-of-towner find a place to park.

At first in his twentieth-century gothic revival office, I felt intimidated by its high ceilings, pointed windows, wood panels, and stonework. In no time at all he put me at ease, and I summarized the 20-minute persuasive talk I had running through my mind. I told him about how my own entheogenic experiences had started me taking religion seriously, how various philosophers of religion, including Huston Smith, thought about them, and how Bob Jesse and I were hoping to organize a scholarly, scientific, and religious conference. CSP hoped the conference would attract recognized, responsible authorities in religion, mental health, and psychology to reopen the door to how entheogens might support spiritual development. I wondered if CTS would agree to co-sponsor such a conference.

I was about to start my longer, more detailed spiel, when Ken said: 'Yes, CTS can co-sponsor the conference' but their support would have to be limited to placing it under CTS's auspices. They couldn't support it financially. I was delighted, and although I had a more detailed pitch to make to Ken, I knew enough to stop a pitch when someone agrees. CSP hadn't expected financial support (Bob Jesse was already looking for private sponsors); just CTS's sponsorship in name. I was delighted. Ken took me to lunch at the Quadrangle Club, the University of Chicago's faculty club. There, I filled him in on some background information on entheogens and our hopes for the conference. His questions were thoughtful, insightful, probing, and always right on the button.

Driving back to DeKalb along Interstate 88 later that afternoon, I realized Ken was much more than a gracious host. He understood that there was more to religion than one church could encompass and, I guess one could say: The Lord works in mysterious ways. Even entheogenic ways. It took me until I wrote *Psychoactive Sacraments'* acknowledgments to get my thoughts in order:

> Thank you, Rev. Kenneth Smith, retired President of Chicago Theological Seminary, and thank you CTS for

co-sponsoring the Vallombrosa Conference-Retreat. By recognizing the social injustice being done to entheogen users and by expressing the spiritual courage to support an unpopular expression of religious exploration, your co-sponsorship made it possible for the Council on Spiritual Practices to attract some of the best minds to this meeting. Personally, I am proud that CTS is a seminary of my denomination, and we are once again in the forefront of human rights as we were in the public schools movement, the founding of universities, abolition, women in the ministry, and sexual orientation. You make me proud to be a Congregationalist-UCC (p. 253).

Had I known it at the time, I would have inserted 'aiding the *Amistad's* crew.' CTS's co-sponsorship meant CSP could approach Huston Smith with the assurance that the conference-retreat would be more than another meeting of people left over from the heady 60s.

One of the conferences' outcomes for me helped me imagine a sort of Tri-Borough Bridge linking peak/mystical experiences, entheogens, and anomalous religious/spiritual healing. The span between the entheogenic uses of psychedelics and mystical experiences was pretty clear in my mind; although, I realize it is still a tenuous span in other people's minds. Huston's outlook echoes Grinspoon and Bakalar's analysis two decades earlier in their comprehensive review of psychedelic research.

> It should not be necessary to supply any more proof that psychedelic drugs produce experiences that those who undergo them regard as religious in the fullest sense.
>
> Lester Grinspoon & James Bakalar
> *Psychedelic Drugs Reconsidered*

In addition, 'drug-induced religious and mystical experience is often reported to be unusually intense.' In support of this assertion, they cite some research by the theologian Walter Clark whose 1974 book *Chemical Ecstasy* was one of the first books on entheogens (before the word was coined, actually).

Walter Clark conducted an experiment in which he gave LSD to eight subjects; nine to eleven months later he asked them to rate the intensity of the experiences on a scale of one to five in various categories. The most common single rating was five — 'beyond anything ever experienced or even imagined' — on measures like timelessness, spacelessness, paradoxicality, presence of God, ultimate reality, blessedness and peace, mystery, and rebirth. As a professor at Andover-Newton Theological School, Clark recruited the seminarians for Pahnke's Good Friday Experiment.

As important as these religious issues and distinctions are, in this chapter we are going to side-step them, and focus instead on entheogen-induced mystical experiences' effects on the immune system. Additional support for the proposition that psychedelics can induce mystical experiences comes from a more recent review. In his 1995 book, *The Facilitation of Religious Experience*, psychologist of religion Ralph Hood judges 'that somewhere between 35 and 50 percent of psychedelic participants report religious experiences of a mystical or numinous nature, even without religious contexts.' This number rises to about 90% if one includes reports with any religious imagery or religious vocabulary. As the designer of the widely-used *Mysticism Scale* and a professor of the psychology of religion at the University of Tennessee at Chattanooga, Hood is one of the most empirically experienced people in describing and evaluating mystical experiences.

The literature abounds with instances of entheogen-occasioned mystical experiences. The next question is: Do these entheogen-occasioned mystical experiences share characteristics with experiences that are known to strengthen the immune system? If so, might psychedelic mystical experiences boost our immune systems, providing a new psychoneuroimmunological path to healing?

Chapter 7

From POTT MUSIC to Spontaneous Remission

In the last chapter we saw that levels of sIgA —salivary immunoglobulin A — rise during positive emotions and fall during negative ones. IgA is one of our immune system's defenses. And we hypothesized that the positive emotions in day-to-day life resemble stronger versions of the overwhelmingly positive feelings that accompany psychedelic mystical experiences. In this chapter we'll explore those relationships in more depth then note that the characteristics they commonly share also commonly appear during spontaneous remission of illnesses. Have we discovered a path from psychedelic mystical experiences to powerful emotions to spontaneous healing — even to spiritual healing?

Characteristics of Mystical Experiences

It's important to distinguish between the different ways that the phrase 'mystical experience' is used in common language and in philosophy and religion. As most people use it in everyday language, 'mystical' brings up images of parapsychology, the occult, cultic practices, and with television shows about 'the unexplained.' In philosophy, religious studies, and the psychology of religion, 'mystical experience' denotes a specific experience or a group of similar experiences. (There is considerable discussion on this point.) Typically, mystical experiences are characterized by subjective qualities. These are: (1) a feeling of oneness — that is, ego transcendence; (2) objectivity and reality — noetic quality or sense of profound truth; (3) a transcendence of time and space; (4) a feeling of sacredness; (5) deeply felt positive mood; (6) an awareness of paradoxicality — an awareness that is anomalous in the Western scientific paradigm; (7) a feeling that the experience is ineffable; (8) transiency — it lasts a short time; and (9) positive changes in attitude and/or behavior. What is particularly interesting about these nine from a healing perspective is that they resemble the subjective characteristics that are also associated with both strengthened salivary IgA levels and with spontaneous remissions. Are we onto something here? After a little mnemonic device to remember them by, we'll look into the possibilities.

POTT MUSIC

Until the fall semester of 2002, I had a hard time remembering these 9 characteristics, so I challenged my *Foundations of Psychedelic Studies* class to come up with a mnemonic device. The class is a Junior Seminar in Northern Illinois University's Honors Program. A mnemonic device is an aide to help remember something, like 'Thirty days has September ...' Having students write mnemonics doesn't just help teach them the content for that mnemonic. They realize they have the power to write mnemonic devices themselves, a learning-how-to-learn skill they can use throughout their lives.

After forming small in-class working groups, we started with the list of characteristics of mystical experiences from Paula Jo Hruby's chapter in my anthology *Psychoactive*

Sacramentals. After brainstorming a bit with her group, Cathy Stresinshe came up with POTT MUSIC.

- **P**aradoxicality — Opposites seem equally true, and violations of natural laws and reason are acceptable.
- **O**bjectivity — Insightful knowledge and illumination seem certain and real. Called a 'noetic' quality.
- **T**ranscendence — Time and/or space are transcended. A sense of spacelessness and/or timelessness.
- **T**ransiency — Duration is limited.
- **M**ood — Deeply felt positive mood: joy, peace, blessedness, love, agapé.
- **U**nity — Either external as in 'All is one' or internal as the self merging with the 'inner world.'
- **S**acredness — A sense of reverence for being in the presence of the divine or holy
- **I**neffability — Difficult or impossible to explain in words. Language is inadequate.
- **C**hange — Behavior and changes in attitudes toward self, others, life, and mystical experience itself. Often accompanied with a redirection of motivation away from ego-centered gains and toward serving humanity and/or cosmic values.

I teach this mnemonic device to my classes each semester. When I want to refreshen my knowledge of mystical experiences, I consult Dr. Hruby's chapter.

Mystical Experiences — Undecided Issues

By providing more examples of mystical experiences to study, psychedelics will also provide information on some contentious questions. People describe mystical experiences in overlapping ways, and there is on-going discussion about whether these experiences are basically one experience that different people and cultures describe differently or whether they are a family of related experiences with important differences between them. With a variety of psychedelics, different kinds of people to take them, and unlimited locations to take them in, careful experimentation when they become legal will help resolve these questions. At least they can make our thinking better informed and more sophisticated.

Until psychedelics' rediscovery in the late 20th Century, these and other questions were for arm-chair philosophers. In the future these religious, philosophical, and psychological arguments will be settled by empirical observations, and will be based on current experiments, not ideological assumptions. Here again is another advance in knowledge that psychedelics provide.

Another set of disagreements is over what characteristics an experience must have to qualify as 'mystical.' One of the real advances of psychedelics is that they give us a way to produce mystical experiences or at least simulate them rather than sitting around waiting for them to happen spontaneously or relying on the small number of times they occurred in past history. Here too, psychedelics advance the study of mystical experiences from arm- chair philosophy and ungrounded theological speculation to experimental psychology. Or should we call it 'experimental philosophy' and 'experimental theology'?

As important and fascinating as they are, in this chapter, we will bypass such discussions about the meanings and characteristics. We'll use a number of terms interchangeably. In this chapter, mystical experiences will be denoted by any of the following experiences: positive feelings of transcendence, self-transcendence, temporary ego-loss, ego-transcendence, unitive consciousness, oneness with the universe, cosmic consciousness, no-self, transpersonal states, divine grace, divine rapture, religious conversion experience, peak experience, mystical unity, and others that POTT MUSIC describes.

A byproduct of studying entheogen-occasioned mystical experiences, though, might be that the reactions of the immune system and other physiological measures will give us clues about the different varieties of mystical experiences. That is, measuring immune responses and other physiological parameters of these events might be one way to categorize the kinds and strengths of mystical experiences.

Effects of Mystical Experiences

Thanks to Ralph Hood's construction of a *Mysticism Scale* in 1975 and its subsequent modifications and thanks to the concurrent growth of transpersonal psychology, there is a substantial amount of empirical research on the effects of mystical experiences. Trying to tell my classes about peak experiences and psychedelically energized mystical experiences lead me to collecting some of this information for a class handout. It is now in Council on Spiritual Practices' website as 'States of Unitive Consciousness: Research Summary.' In 1988 David Lukoff and Frances Lu compiled most of the research on mystical experiences for 'Transpersonal Psychology Research Review. Topic Mystical Experiences.' an article in the *Journal of Transpersonal Psychology*. Since then Lu and Lukoff have published more on this topic. In 1966 Dr. Hruby's dissertation *The Varieties of Mystical Experience, Spiritual Practices, and Psychedelic Drug Use Among College Students* summarized the research on mystical states. The reviews of all of these authors support the connection between mystical experiences and mental health, a key link in the Emxis hypothesis.

What do they say? To begin, these summaries show that mystical experiences tend to be associated with indicators of positive mental health. Further, as compared with people who have not had mystical experiences, those who have experienced them report lives that are more meaningful and hopeful and more often report that they feel a purpose or direction in their lives. They have higher levels of education and income and rate themselves higher in levels of personal talent and capabilities, self-sufficiency, intelligence, and ego strength. They picture themselves as more psychologically mature, less motivated by personal fame and a desire for high income, and as more altruistic. They say their mystical experiences were more conducive to mental health than to mental illness.

Now, because most of these findings come from correlational studies, it is not clear whether mystical experiences help produce these characteristics, intensify already existing traits, or occur because of a third factor such as personality traits. Future experimental studies with entheogens might help clear up this ambiguity. In any event, for us the critical question in this chapter is whether the characteristics of mystical experiences are associated with improved functioning of the immune system.

The Immune System and Salivary Immunoglobulin A

In my own experience, mystical experiences certainly feel healthy. Remember: I am not saying that all psychedelic experiences are mystical ones, only the ones that meet the POTT MUSIC criteria. Physically I feel: 'This is what it feels like to be truly and deeply healthy.' Needless tension melts away. I feel that my blood is flowing into parts of my body where its flow was restricted before, places I hold tension, especially my shoulders and upper back. My breathing is smoother, deeper, and easier. I imagine — or am I actually feeling it? — that I can feel more oxygen moving into my blood stream. In a sense it is relaxing just as a sound sleep is, but, of course, I am awake. My hands, where I also hold tension, relax. And to my surprise the first time it happened, I not only felt more flexible, but could get into yoga positions that I couldn't in my ordinary awake state. After my sessions, the flexibility remains for a day or two, but then I head back toward my normal restricted range of movement. Do these positive emotions, bodily feelings, and thoughts accompany a healthier body?

If so, this increased health should show up in my immune system, and in this section we will focus specifically on increased levels of salivary IgA — sIgA — as a presumed indicator of overall immune strength. Salivary IgA is, of course, only one measure of immune function. I select it for its many advantages. Other immune indicators presumably could show similar effects and deserve attention too.

Medical researchers H. B Valdimarsdottir and A. A. Stone describe IgA this way: IgA 'is the major immunoglobulin in the fluids that bathe the mucosal surfaces of the body and the surfaces that are the paths of entry to invading bacteria and viruses into the body (e.g. tears, saliva, gastrointestinal, vaginal, nasal, and bronchial secretions)', because one of its locations is saliva in the mouth, IgA is relatively easy to sample. With some care on how the sample is taken and the amount taken, a simple swab in the mouth will do it. It isn't necessary to take a blood sample or break the skin.

I hope this chapter will encourage qualified researchers to study positive emotional experiences induced by entheogens by taking IgA samples before psychedelic sessions, during them, and afterwards. Salivary IgA has the advantage of being obtainable quickly while causing a minimum of interruption to an on-going entheogenic session. A minimally intrusive mouth swab would be easily appropriate during a situation when suggestibility is heightened and subjects may be easily frightened or stressed by blood-taking procedures. And these could well be beyond the professional qualifications and personal preferences of potential researchers into this area, including theologians and sociologists.

Another reason for using salivary measures, and specifically IgA, as indicators of the immune system's health is the large number of studies that form a theoretical and empirical base for doing so. Some of these studies examine IgA at many sites in our bodies. Others look only for salivary IgA. In their 1992 review *Saliva as a Diagnostic Fluid*, Glock, Heller, and Malamud listed 2298 citations from over 7500 that they initially retrieved. Of these, 174 consider immunoglobulins. From 1993 through January 2004, *Medline*, the major online research base of the National Library of Medicine, listed 496 published studies. Although many of them looked at physical stress, few of them looked at emotional state. Thus, in all, salivary IgA studies are embedded in a widely recognized research base with established methods and professional practices but with little attention to positive emotions and desirable outcomes.

From the perspective of the Emxis hypothesis, a problem with sIgA studies done so far is that only a small fraction address wellness, positive health, or positive experiences. However, if we assume that positive emotions have the reverse effect of negative emotions, the Emxis hypothesis is supported by a large database of illness-related studies which show that stressors reduce salivary IgA and other immune functions.

A final reason to focus on salivary IgA is that there are some intriguing research leads that link stressful daily events in one's life with lower salivary IgA levels and positive events with higher levels. For example, a series of studies by A. A. Stone and others found desirable and undesirable daily events influence IgA up or down respectively, and as the Emxis hypothesis assumes, mood mediates the effects. We shall return to these studies.

Psychospiritual and psychosocial boosts for the immune system

Might mystical experiences (peak experiences) connect entheogens and increased immune system functioning? If mystical experiences share characteristics with events that enhance salivary IgA, it is entirely reasonable to suppose that they could make these links.

Stress reduction

We need to keep in mind that most research has studied salivary IgA and stress reduction. Most studies so far reduce negative emotions rather than increase positive ones. This is in keeping with contemporary medicine's orientation to curing illness rather enhancing wellness. Coping with negative mood may not be the same as increasing positive mood, especially increasing positive mood to the great extremes occurring during some mystical experiences. Nevertheless, the reduction of unpleasant emotions, depression, and other stressful daily events that weaken the immune system as measured in essence do increase in positive moods.

In 'Psychosocial Factors and Secretory Immunoglobulin A', Valdimarsdottir and Stone select and summarize about two dozen research studies on the relationships between sIgA and both stressful events and stress-reduction interventions. Although the authors caution that 'methodological refinements are needed before more definitive conclusions can be made,' they maintain that the studies indicate that various stress-reduction interventions are associated with increases in salivary IgA levels. But do the interventions that increase salivary IgA resemble mystical experiences? If so, we have a hint — by no means strong evidence — that mystical experiences (non-psychedelic or psychedelic) may help our immune systems too.

Among the stress-reduction techniques that boost the immune system, Valdimarsdottir and her colleagues list:

the relaxation response, progressive relaxation, guided visualization, imaging powerful immune functions, back massage, music combined with self-induced state of appreciation. David McClelland and his co-researchers found that self-hypnosis, suggestions, and humorous movies help our immune systems too. By a wonderful ironic twist, the person who lead this study is the same McClelland who hired Timothy Leary and later fired him.

> McClelland poured us both more wine. He lit another stogie. 'Okay, I'm prepared to offer you a job at Harvard.'
> 'Are you serious?'
> 'I'm intrigued.' said Professor McClelland. 'There's no question that what you're advocating is going to be the future of American psychology. You're not a lone voice. There are several hotshots in our profession — like Benjamin Spock, Carl Rogers, Abraham Maslow, Harry Stack Sullivan, Milton Gloaming — urging that we emphasize inner potential and personal growth through self-reliance, so patients avoid dependence on authoritarian doctors and dogmas. You're spelling out front-line tactics. You're just what we need to shake things up at Harvard.'
>
> Timothy Leary
> *Flashbacks* (p. 18)

What do these stress reduction techniques have to do with mystical experiences? They are consistent with the decreased need for ego defensiveness that accompanies ego-transcendent states. They also portray feelings of belonging and unity, deeply felt positive mood. And these are all characteristics of mystical experiences too. If we assume that human abilities vary in strength from one mindbody state to another as Chapters 8–14 contend, it is likely that visualization, suggestion, hypnosis, and imaging are more powerful in some altered states of consciousness. And these cognitive processes are often powerful during instances of unusual healing. Do psychedelics produce states of consciousness where these abilities are stronger? We'll pick up this idea below as we look at spontaneous remission.

In short, although IgA studies do not directly investigate the hypothetical relationship between mystical states and improved immune function, as a whole they are in the expected direction. Perhaps these stress-reduction interventions can best be considered as mild examples of more powerful entheogenic interventions. The most common feature of both types of interventions is positive emotions.

Social support

Studies of social support offer another possible link to the characteristics of mystical experiences. For example, the article 'Academic Stress, Social Support, and Secretory Immunoglobulin A,' which appeared in *Journal of Personality and Social Psychology* in 1988, found that high levels of IgA in the saliva are associated with social support. For people who have had a mystical experience, do the feelings of unity, belonging in the universe, and 'coming to one's ultimate home' provide feelings of extreme support, even cosmic support? Here again, the hypothesis is tantalizing, but the data missing. For people who have experienced these states, cosmic belonging may substitute – more than substitute – for ordinary, interpersonal social support.

Studies of social support, positive psychological mood, and desirable daily events show all three are correlated with increased salivary IgA. These studies also provide some general support for the Emxis hypothesis, especially the link between positive experience and increased IgA in the saliva. They are at least consistent with this hypothesis.

So far what have we shown? First, psychedelics sometimes produce mystical experiences. Mystical experiences
and positive emotional experiences that strengthen the
immune system resemble each other in several vital characteristics. These connections are *sometimes*, *partial*, and
perhaps. They aren't solidly established. This leaves us
with the questions: Do mystical experiences strengthen
the immune system too? And: Do entheogen energized
mystical experiences boost the immune system? If we
could discover some instances of healing occurring
because of — or associated with — mystical states, our
chain of reasoning and the Emxis hypothesis would gain
support, although still not be solidly proven.

Mystical states and spontaneous remission

Let's ratchet up the importance of the possible significance of
the Emxis hypothesis. If positive day-to-day experiences
strengthen the immune system somewhat, might powerfully positive experiences — mystical states, states of unitive
consciousness, or ego-transcendent states — strengthen
the immune system a great deal? Do we find instances of
mystical experiences being connected with unusual cures?
Some suggestive data supports this supposition.

In *Spontaneous Remission: An Annotated Bibliography*,
Brendan O'Regan and Carlyle Hirshberg present a table of
'Psychospiritual Correlates of Remission.' They resemble
both the POTT MUSIC characteristics of mystical experiences, and the daily events, positive moods, and upbeat
attitudes that increase levels of sIgA. In their list of 27 correlates of spontaneous remission, we find our mood-
enhancing friends which boost sIgA.

- group support
- hypnosis/suggestion
- meditation
- relaxation techniques

- mental imagery
- psychotherapy/psychoanalysis
- behavioral therapy
- group therapy
- miraculous spiritual phenomena
- prayer/spiritual belief
- religious/spiritual conversion
- autonomous behavior/increased autonomy
- faith/positive outcome expectancy
- a fighting spirit
- denial
- lifestyle/attitude/behavioral (changes)
- social relationships/interpersonal relationship/family support
- positive emotions/acceptance of negative emotions
- environmental/social awareness/altruistic
- expression of needs/demands/self-nurturing
- sense of control/internal locus of control
- desire/will to live
- increased or altered sensory perception
- taking responsibility for the illness
- sense of purpose
- placebo effect
- diet/exercise.

These accompany spontaneous remission, and some of them are clear instances of the POTT MUSIC traits of mystical experiences. Others look like emotional, social, religious. and psychological cousins.

Once again, coincidences in my personal life informed my professional interest in the Emxis idea. *Spontaneous Remission* was published by the Institute of Noetic Sciences. Remember: the feeling of a noetic sense of knowing — objectivity — with its deep feeling of truth and understanding is one of the characteristics of mystical experiences. IONS was founded by one of my former professors at Stanford, Willis Harman, and by the astronaut Edgar Mitchell. Mitchell apparently had a noetic experience during his trip in outer space. It's easy to imagine someone floating weightless in space with much sensory input cut off having a mystical experience.

At Stanford I was writing my dissertation on Abraham Maslow's needs hierarchy and heard that Willis Harman, a professor in the School of Engineering, was studying Maslow at the Stanford Research Institute, so I wanted to meet him to find out what he knew. At that time Stanford Research Institute was associated with Stanford University, but Stanford later spun it off to become the independent SRI.

At that point, I had no interest in psychedelics, just Maslow's ideas. Although that included his work on peak experiences, my interest was limited to his needs hierarchy … at least until I took Willis Harman's signature course. He taught a little seminar limited to graduate students. It was titled *The Human Potential* and was in a department called — of all things — Engineering Economic Systems. The course was so popular it had a waiting list of two quarters to get in. I signed up and waited.

Two quarters went by, and I was sitting around a table with about 2 dozen other graduate students from departments all over Stanford. The course focused on unusual human abilities, including some that were on the fringes of academic respectability such as parapsychological abilities and meditation. In the late 1960s just as physiological research on meditation was getting started, an academic interest in meditation was seen as foolish and raised questions about one's gullibility and professionalism.

One day in class a graduate student couple described their first psychedelic experience the previous weekend. They were saying good things about their experience! This didn't fit in with what I had been taught about these nasty, brain-rotting drugs. Yet they seemed sane enough, and it was clear they valued their experience in ways that were difficult to describe, maybe impossible. In spite of what I had learned from TV and newspapers, they seemed to have benefited from their LSD session. Some other students in the class nodded understandingly, congratulated them. A discussion ensued about these experiences and left me far behind. What under the sun were they talking about? I knew my fellow classmates well enough to know they were logical, bright, inquisitive, graduate students at Stanford. How could so many of them have had psychedelic experiences and not be locked away in some loony bin?

Again good luck struck. One of my classmates had purchased a series of tickets for a program called 'Esalen at Stanford.' Esalen Institute, a parent of the growth center movement that was burgeoning in the late 60s and early 70s, was expensive for students to go to, so Esalen arranged to bring their leaders to Stanford for a series of weekend workshops and lectures. My classmate friend couldn't attend one weekend and gave me his ticket. Good luck doubled up. The weekend was a series of lectures by Alan Watts, a British-born and educated priest-scholar-Christian-Buddhist. His topic was psychedelics and spiritual transformation. I had no idea who this guy was, but our class discussion about psychedelics piqued my curiosity.

I attended the lectures. This erudite speaker's lectures combined spiritual development, Eastern and Christian views of the human mind (also a new topic for me), and psychedelics. I was blown away. Although these topics were in the air in the late 60s, all these topics were ones I hadn't heard discussed in a serious academic way before. I wasn't convinced by what Watts said, but I realized this was an area I knew nothing about and one I became curious about.

When Willis Harman retired from Stanford to co-found the Institute of Noetic Sciences, I was one of the first members and kept up on new ideas about the human potential through IONS' bulletins.

Another interesting fact about IONS is the word *noetic* in its name. The noetic sense is the feeling of 'realer than real' and profound knowledge that sometimes occurs during mystical experiences. Not only is it a characteristic of direct knowing, but the word's Greek root (*nous*) is linked to that of *Gnostics*, the early Christian believers who lost the power struggle with what became mainstream Christianity. Our word *know* is another language cousin. Appropriately enough: the motto of the college I attended, Hamilton College, is one of the precepts from the Greek oracle at ancient Delphi — ΓΝΩΘΙ ΣΕΑΥΤΟΝ — Gnothi Seauton — in English letters. It means 'Know Thyself.' Furthermore, researchers have recently found out that the women oracles at Delphi — the Pythia — went into altered states of consciousness to reach their knowledge (their gnosis, their noetic knowing) by inhaling psychoactive fumes that were emitted from a crack in the earth.

In the early part of the Christian era, the successful Christian group which won the interchurch power struggle to become mainstream selected which books would become the collection we now call the *Bible*. The Gnostic books were excluded. But Gnostic texts are making a comeback largely through the work of Elaine Pagels, a professor of religion at Princeton. Coincidentally enough, she grew up on the Stanford campus where her father was a professor. As she points out, according to the Gnostic gospels, spiritual awakening can come to anyone through their own visions; everyone can have direct access to God, and Jesus' resurrection represents a spiritual transformation that is open to everyone. These are the claims that entheogenists make too.

Bang! Here we are back to considering psychoactive sacramentals and their role producing mystical experiences, boosting spiritual intelligence, and advancing spiritual transformation. To investigate this possible connection, we need to know: Are there significant similarities between mystical experiences and spontaneous remissions?

Many of the 27 psychospiritual correlates of spontaneous healing that Brendan O'Regan and Carlyle Hirshberg found are characteristics of both mystical experiences and events that boost salivary IgA. Others, such as sense of belonging, discarding ego-centeredness, reorienting one's life, and altered states of consciousness are typical of mystical experiences but do not appear in salivary IgA research — yet. The correlates that emphasize insights into one's personal life and social relationships parallel the results of decreased ego-attachment that often follow ego transcendence, both psychedelic and non-psychedelic. One cluster of correlates is composed of experiences of altered-states phenomena — the very nature of mystical experience.

To me it seems reasonable to suppose that the persistent cluster of feelings, thoughts, moods, and behaviors that occur during mystical experiences, IgA-boosting daily events, and spontaneous remission could be intensified by powerful psychedelic mystical experiences.

At this point, an inclination toward a positive answer can be only a surmise. O'Regan and Hirshberg report disappointingly few findings that show a relationship between mystical states and unaccountable cures. Given that spontaneous remissions and mystical experiences both occur at low rates in a population, this may not be so surprising. Still, *Spontaneous Remission* provides suggestive anecdotal and clinical observations.

Ego-transcendence

The authors note that at the first conference on spontaneous regression held at the Johns Hopkins University in
1974, as reported in *Medical World News*: 'Dr. Renee
Mastrovito of the neuropsychiatric service at Memorial
Sloan Kettering Cancer Center alluded to historical refer-
ences to cures following religious conversion or prayer.'
They also point to a study of five selected cases 'who made
a narrow escape from cancer,' by Ikemi and 3 other Japa-
nese researchers in 1975. According to O'Regan and
Hirshberg, these authors claim that the patients' spontaneous cures were 'supported and encouraged by their religious faith or favorable change of human environment
[social relationship]' and suggest 'that the background of
Oriental thought also might help them reach such a blessed
state of mind.' In three of the five cases, 'the unchanged or
rather elevated immunological capacity which was usually
lowered in cancer patients has been confirmed.'

A 1983 the *American Society of Psychosomatic Dentistry
and Medicine Journal* reported on a survey of 18 cases of
cancer regression. This survey by C. Weinstock notes the
typical feelings of hope, purpose, and meaning that follow
mystical experiences: 'All 18 definitely did not have anything for which to live before the favorable psychosocial
change, and all found life very much worth living afterwards.' Here again, these are not hard tests of the idea that
the Emxis hypothesis leads us to expect, but they are hints
in the expected direction.

O'Regan and Hirshberg also cite clinical reports by
Meares of 12 cases of spontaneous regression of cancers
associated with intensive meditation. In the discussion of
one case, Meares wrote: 'It may well be that the extreme
reduction of anxiety in these patients triggers off the
mechanism which becomes active in the rare spontaneous
remissions. This would be consistent with the observation
that spontaneous remissions are often associated with

some kind of religious experience or profound psychological reaction.' Sacredness, unity, ego-transcendence, positive mood: these can be triggered by mystical experiences,
psychedelic or not.

We can suppose that the religious conversion experiences, blessed states of mind, and marked favorable
psychosocial change reported in the studies above probably indicate strongly felt positive moods and possibly
peak or ego-transcendent mystical experiences. From a
transpersonal perspective, a consistent source of psychological anxiety and its resulting physical stress is over-
identification with the ego. As the saying goes: The ego
has problems: the ego is a problem. Might it be that ego
transcendence or dis-identification during meditation or
in other ways helps account for instances of spontaneous
remission?

Ego transcendence is also a common experience during
intense psychedelic sessions. While using psychedelics
with cancer patients not to cure cancer but as an adjunct to
psychotherapy, William Richards, an ordained Methodist
minister now working as a psychotherapist, reported that
the most significant variable in psychedelic psychotherapy is 'the peak experience variable.'

Taking Up Unfinished Work

In their summary of psychosocial factors effecting sIgA,
Drs. Valdimarsdottir and Stone conclude that both negative and positive emotions link daily events and sIgA levels. This 'indicates that researchers should not only focus
on the role of negative affect but should also consider the
contribution of positive affect.' The Emxis hypothesis
might add, 'Especially extremely powerful positive affect!'

Twenty-five years ago in *Psychedelic Drugs Reconsidered*,
the book-length review of the scientific and scholarly literature (over 1000 studies), Grinspoon and Bakalar summarized their position:

After more than ten years of almost total neglect, it is time to take up the work that was laid down unfinished in the sixties. We need to arrange a way for people to take psychedelic drugs responsibly under appropriate guidance within the law, and a way for those who want to administer them to volunteers for therapeutic and general research to do so.

They wrote this after examining and compiling nearly all the writing on psychedelic research in psychotherapy, religion, creativity, psychology, and related fields.

Now, two and a half decades later, little progress has been made, but the Emxis hypothesis gives another rationale to restart this research: Entheogen-induced mystical experiences may boost the immune system. Here is a project to link medicine, religion, and psychology.

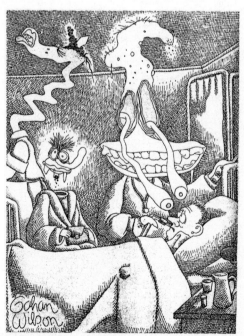

'Now those pills you just took may produce some visual side effects.' Reproduced by special permission of *Playboy Magazine*, Copyright © 1982 by Playboy

PART 3

Multistate Mind

Some years ago I myself made some observations on this aspect of nitrous oxide intoxication and reported them in print. One conclusion was forced upon my mind at that time, and my impression of its truth has ever remained unshaken. It is that our normal waking consciousness, rational consciousness as we call it, is but one special type of consciousness, whilst all about it, parted from it by the filmiest of screens, there lie potential forms of consciousness entirely different. We may go through life without suspecting their existence; but apply the requisite stimulus, and at a touch they are there in all completeness, definite types of mentality which probably somewhere have their field of application and adaptation. No account of the universe in its totality can be final which leaves these other forms of consciousness quite disregarded. How to regard them is the question, — for they are so discontinuous with ordinary consciousness. Yet they may determine attitudes though they cannot furnish formulas, and open a region through which they fail to give a map. At any rate, they forbid a premature closing of our accounts with reality.

William James
Varieties of Religious Experience
(p. 298, Mentor edition, 1958)

Chapter 8

Bigger, Stronger, Brighter
A New Relationship with our Minds

One of the delightful things about psychedelics was discovering their implications for how we think about our minds. (Remember: I'm an intuitive thinking type who thrives on looking at the big-picture, theoretical implications of things.) While Aldous Huxley's *The Doors of Perception* brilliantly describes some of psychedelics' effects, and Huston Smith's *Cleansing the Doors of Perception* looks at some of the implications of psychedelics for religion and spiritual development, I'd have to say I am fascinated by 'the doors of conception.' What psychedelics teach us about our minds intrigues me. Our minds are larger than we had previously supposed. They have abilities beyond those of our ordinary state. And as we develop our minds' fullest potentials, we'll learn new ways to become intelligent: we are brighter than we think.

Psychedelics as Psychomagnifiers

The general approach to psychedelics is to consider them 'unspecific amplifiers of our minds,' to use Stan Grof's phrase. Like a microscope to our minds, we can experience and observe its contents in greater detail. Handy parallels come from medicine and astronomy. Modern biology and medicine would be impossible without the magnifying abilities of the microscope: first the optical microscope, then the electron microscope. Using these magnifying instruments, we have detailed maps (atlases) of, say, the liver or kidney; we know things about these organs that were unknown before microscopes were invented. Modern biology and medicine would be impossible without them.

At the present time I consider LSD to be a powerful unspecific amplifier or catalyst of biochemical and physiological processes in the brain. ... The capacity of LSD and some other psychedelic drugs to exteriorize otherwise invisible phenomena and processes and make them the subject of scientific investigation gives these substances a unique potential as diagnostic instruments and research tools for the exploration of the human mind. It does not seem inappropriate and exaggerated to compare their significance for psychiatry and psychology to that of the microscope for medicine or the telescope for astronomy.

Stanislav Grof
Realms of the Human Unconscious
(pp. 32–3)

Similarly, the optical telescope opened new realms of the heavens for direct observation, and as a result our views of cosmology and creation changed. Thanks to radio telescopes and telescopes located on satellites above our earth's atmosphere, we are extending our knowledge even further. Astronomy, astrophysics, and cosmology will never be the same.

When we think of psychedelics as 'psychomagnifiers' — doing for our minds what the microscope did for medicine and the telescope did for astronomy — the natural questions arise: What does a detailed map of our minds look like? And: What will future mind explorers discover? To piece together our new atlases of our body and of the sky, biologists and astronomers are assembling an enormous number of individual pieces into overall jigsaw puzzles. For an enlarged map of our minds, Stan Grof has assembled thousands of individual mind-snapshots into a map that he presents in *Realms of the Human Unconscious* and some of his subsequent books. With particular emphasis on the emotional aspects of our minds, the psychedelic technique for mapping our minds and Grof's map offer advances in psychology and psychotherapy that may eventually parallel the advances that microscopes brought to medicine and telescopes to astronomy.

Besides mapping our minds, psychedelics provide new ways to do psychotherapy. They can help produce creative solutions to problems. They have stimulated new directions in the arts, and they even promise to strengthen spiritual intelligence. But if we step back for a moment from the psychomagnifying aspects of psychedelics, they exemplify a broader insight into how we can study our minds and eventually how we can develop them to their fullest extent — how we can become fully educated. This insight comes when we recognize that our minds do useful work in mindbody states in addition to our ordinary, awake state. This is the idea of the multistate mind.

In my course *Foundations of Psychedelic Studies* at Northern Illinois University, I find the following imaginary dialog is a good way to teach this point:

Imagine that a friend of ours has just bought a powerful new computer and is telling us about it.

'What are you going to use it for?' I ask.

'I'm going to play chess with it,' he answers.

'Are you going to use it to write, check your spelling, and use the thesaurus?' you ask.

'No,' he responds, 'I'm going to play chess.'

Another friend asks, 'You're going to send email, aren't you? You can communicate around the world on the Internet and find information on the World Wide Web.'

'No!' he insists, 'I'm going to play chess!'

'What about bookkeeping, spreadsheets, and tracking your financial records?' asks another friend who is an accountant. 'You're going to use it for these, aren't you?'

'NO! NO!' our friend shouts angrily, 'I'm going to play chess!'

We would all recognize that our friend is underutilizing a powerful information-processing resource. He can use many programs. He doesn't have to limit himself to the chess program.

In the ways we use our minds — rather in the ways we don't use them— we resemble our chess-playing friend. Just as a computer has many different information processing programs, and certain ones are good for their specific purposes, our minds are similar to computers. They have many information processing programs too, each with its own purposes. For our minds these 'programs' are our various mindbody states, also called 'states of consciousness.' On pages 218-219, I explain why I prefer to call them 'mindbody states' rather than 'states of consciousness.' Like our chess-playing friend, we unnecessarily restrict ourselves to using only our ordinary awake mindbody state, which is just one of many useful mental programs.

The Program-State Analogy

programs : computers :: mindbody states : minds

We stunt ourselves, our children, and the human future by educating only one mental state — one cognitive processing program. This chapter focuses on a wide, multistate view of our minds. Chapters 9–14 look at some of the implications of this view.

The Singlestate Fallacy

Psychology and education systematically exclude vast fields of information about other mindbody states. I call this error in thinking *'The Singlestate Fallacy'. The Singlestate Fallacy is the erroneous assumption that all worthwhile abilities reside in our normal, awake mindbody state.* Chess is not the only game in town. If education and psychology are to be realistic about the human mind, they must recognize its multistate nature.

In the last three decades the singlestate fallacy has been undermined by five interlocking sets of ideas: altered states psychology, transpersonal psychology, mindbody medicine, anthropology, and the philosophy of consciousness.

I hope you won't misunderstand what I'm implying. I'm not denigrating our ordinary, normal state. I'm a real fan of our usual, awake state. I spend most of my time in it, and I do most of my work in it, sometimes altered by cups of tea or chocolate. Limited as it is, it's a fine state, and I expect it has evolved as our psychological home base for good reasons. I'm in it as I write this, and I use it most of the time day-in and day-out. It's a fine and valuable state with untapped potentials. What I hope you'll understand is that other states have their uses too. It's our single-minded (pardon the pun) attachment to our usual state that I deplore.

I realize we value sleep and dreaming too, but most people see them primarily as necessary aides to our ordinary state, a sort of servant role in which our ordinary state is still king. There may be interesting leads to our fullest mental development here, though. If sleep and dreams help out our ordinary state, we are seeing how one state can benefit from other states. Is this a clue? Since sleeping and dreaming help our ordinary awake state function well, have we stumbled across a more general principle? Do different mindbody states, properly developed, strengthen and support each other? Meditators, practitioners of the martial arts, and people who use concentrative prayer, for example, report that their regular exercises in these psychotechnologies also aid them in their awake state, in sleep, and even when dreaming. Major unexplored topics are how one state affects others, how they communicate, and other interstate interactions.

We certainly know that some states are detrimental to others. Alcoholism and addiction are clear negative examples, and we don't seem to have any problem accepting that. But we spend less time and effort paying attention to how various states might cross-benefit each other. Odd.

For me and many of my psychedelic colleagues and friends, it was our experiences with psychedelics that opened the multistate door, helping us realize there was much more to our minds than our ordinary awake state. Other people have entered this idea via other doors: meditation, dreams, anesthetics, stimulants, and so forth. Psychedelics certainly aren't the only passageway, but they are so powerful and so overwhelming that one simply can't ignore them. For hundreds of thousands of people, perhaps millions, psychedelics provide first-hand evidence that there's more to mental abilities than we had ever dreamed of. When you finish this book, I hope you'll have a broader take on whatever mental topics most interest you: thinking, emotions, memory, performance, intelligence, and so forth.

Why shouldn't you put LSD in your friend's coffee?

There certainly are less risky ways than psychedelics for exploring our many mindstates. This would be another good time to reread the 'Psychedelic Warning label' near the front of this book. In one of the earliest class meetings of my *Foundations of Psychedelic Studies* class each semester, I point out the dangers of unsupervised, informal psychedelic use by asking this rhetorical question: In addition to being illegal, why shouldn't you put LSD (or other drugs) in your friend's coffee? Of course, the answers apply to themselves too.

- The drugs you buy from a dealer may not actually be the drug you want, and some dealers will sell you anything and tell you it's what you want. Also, its dose is unknown, and it may be contaminated with other drugs or who-knows-what. Unfortunately, this danger is largely a result of our current drug policies.

- Psychedelics can activate parts of your unconscious mind that cause great anxiety and should be faced only in the company of a qualified therapist. These might include traumatic experiences, for example, or childhood fears. Stan Grof's work gives examples of this; fortunately, his patients were undergoing psychedelic psychotherapy not taking the drug on their own. For someone who is prepsychotic, this could cause a bad trip or even tip the balance into psychosis. Normal people can still bring up irrational fears and thoughts that can continue to interfere with their lives after the drug is gone.

- People have idiosyncratic and genetic-based reactions to drugs. Some people are allergic to aspirin, others to antibiotics.

- Genetic differences probably play a role too. For example, Ecstasy (MDMA) works by flooding the space between cells (the synapse) with serotonin. Serotonin is then carried back to the cells by 'transporter proteins' to be reused. Some Ecstasy users are prone to depression because they have a short version of a less efficient gene that produces the transporter. People with 2 short genes are even more susceptible to depression after MDMA. As the field of pharmacogenomics — the study of the interactions between genes and drugs — grows, it's likely that other gene-based drug effects will be discovered. You don't know about your friend's possible reactions to an unknown drug, and your friend probably doesn't know either.

- If your friend is pregnant, psychedelics can instigate a miscarriage by causing uterine contractions. According to Grof's work, if a woman re-experiences the perinatal stage of her own birth, this sometimes induces her own uterus to contract.

- Grof makes a sensitive psychiatric point: Although the myth of psychedelics causing birth defects is fading away, a certain number of babies are born with defects even to mothers who have had excellent prenatal care. If this happens to a mother who did psychedelics when she was pregnant — even though she knows the birth defect rumor is a myth — she doesn't need to think everyday for the rest of her life, 'What if I hadn't?'

- Finally, if you believe as I do, that each person has the right to determine what goes on in his or her own mind, then putting a drug in your friend's coffee destroys this freedom. You are infringing this right to mental self- control.

Extending the Human Mind

My psychedelic colleagues and I have found that once we started thinking with a multistate view, the old singlestate paradigm fades to gray. Without my own psychedelic-based experiences, I doubt I would even have understood this multistate view of our minds and the roads that mindbody psychotechnologies — both psychedelic and non-psychedelic — offer toward our fullest use of our minds. Not only are the experiences themselves important, but they've lead me to read and study other psycho-technologies — other programs for developing our minds. I don't at all think it's an exaggeration to say that for me experiencing psychedelics and following up the intellec-tual avenues they pointed toward were at least the equiva-lent of earning my doctorate at Stanford.

Multistate Assumptions

For me and for some of my psychedelic colleagues, our experiences with psychedelics have helped us expand our assumptions (to what we think are more accurate and real-istic assumptions) about our minds. There are other, safer methods for discovering the experiences that support multistate assumptions too. Some people have reached these conclusions through their direct experiences by yoga, meditation, biofeedback, hypnosis, dream-work, or other mindbody psychotechnologies. Still others know about these ideas through reading or television programs.

Summary

Our minds and their education go far beyond what most people suppose. However, if you are familiar with Eastern psychologies or the state-of-consciousness thread of West-ern psychologies, this book will present some ideas you're already familiar with. Many people have studied various kinds of meditation, dreaming, lucid dreaming, the mar-tial arts, and so forth, but they usually see these as sepa-

A Comparison of Singlestate and Multistate Paradigms

— General Assumptions —

SINGLESTATE ASSUMPTIONS	MULTISTATE ASSUMPTIONS
Human Nature	
Mindbody states other than our ordinary state are interesting curiosities, but of little professional or practical interest.	A significant human trait is the ability to produce and use a variety of mindbody states.
Reality	
Time, space and matter are real. Only experiences in our usual MBS are real.	The experiences of time, space, and matter depend on the MBS in which they are experienced.
Intellectual Climate	
Altered MBSs are not worthy of serious intellectual attention.	The major intellectual error of our times is the failure to recognize the fundamental primacy of mindbody states.
Personal Existence	
A person exists within a material body, in a specific place, and at particular times.	Personal existence may go beyond the usual limits of body-based identity, time, and space.
Knowledge	
All knowledge comes through sense perception and reason.	Reason and perception differ from one MBS to another.

Note: In the above table, MBS is an abbreviation for 'mindbody state.' If you think that these are somewhat unfair characterizations, please remember that such is the nature of ideal types; they fit to varying degrees.

rate topics, isolated from each other. In this book, I hope you'll see that they are all important pieces of a wider, multistate view that integrates them all. On a more organizational level, I hope that some day there will be companies, health services, mind-development centers, and religious orders which will screen applicants for psychedelic sessions, prepare them, guide the sessions, and follow-up people who have had these experiences.

This chapter and the next 4 consider the main questions of mind studies and education:

• What is the nature of the human mind?

• What are its fullest and most beneficial potentials?

• How do we achieve this?

As this chapter claimed, a complete answer to the first question has to include the fact that our minds can achieve and use many mindbody states. Chapter 9, 'The Multistate Paradigm,' sketches a set of ideas I've found useful in thinking about the multistate nature of our minds. I say 'sketch' because much more elaboration needs to be done to fill out this theory. 'Intelligence, Creativity, Meta-intelligence,' Chapter 10, points out how psychedelics and other mindbody psychotechnologies, wisely used, can improve our thinking. Chapter 11, 'Psychology, Science, and Survival' describes some advantages — both in theory and human adaptability — a multistate theory has over a singlestate theory. The title of Chapter 12 'The Major Intellectual Opportunity of Our Times,' speaks for itself.

In Chapters 13 and 14, we'll turn to education. 'It Means Something Different to be Well Educated' and 'Enlarging Learning' show what happens when we transcend the singlestate fallacy's restrictions on mind development. They layout the first steps toward a systematic program for how we might begin to answer, 'What are our minds' fullest and most beneficial potentials?' and 'How do we achieve this?' 'Is the Reprogrammable Brain Adaptigenic?', Chapter 15, looks beyond today's horizons and speculates about 'The Day After Tomorrow's Horizons'.

Chapter 9

The Multistate Paradigm

The multistate paradigm recognizes that our minds and bodies can produce and use many mindbody states. These are sometimes called 'psychophysiological states' or 'states of consciousness.' Because of the many confusing and ambiguous meanings of the word 'consciousness,' I prefer the word *mindbody*. (See pages 218–219.)

When a new view of the human mind appears, it sets off a domino cascade in ideas downstream from it. Realizing that we can produce and use many mindbody states is one of those first-domino ideas. It reconstructs our ideas about what our minds are, how they work, their capabilities, and their cultivation. As a step toward delineating how the multistate paradigm contrasts with the singlestate paradigm, in my 1989 article 'Multistate Education: Metacognitive Implications of the Mindbody Psychotechnologies,' I compared 35 psychological and educational concepts, here adapted to five tables: General Intellectual Assumptions (which is in the previous chapter), Cognition (in Chapter 10), Major Psychologies (in Chapter 11), Learning (in Chapter 13), and Counselling and Mental Health (in Chapter 14). Because we use our minds in all scholarly, intellectual, scientific, and artistic endeavors as well as in practical matters, when our ideas about our mind changes, these all change too.

The three central ideas of the multistate paradigm are (a) mindbody state, (b) mindbody psychotechnologies, and (c) residency. By understanding these concepts in psychedelic states, I've found my appreciation of the infinite human potential greatly expanded.

Mindbody State

Derived from Charles Tart's many works, I define 'mindbody state' as 'an overall pattern of physiological and mental functioning at any one time.' Mind and body (considered as a united whole) produces a large number of states. As shown in the chess analogy in the last chapter, our ordinary awake state is one instance, one 'mental program,' so to speak. In addition to this state, other states are sleep, dreams, meditative states, those states brought about by exercise and spiritual routines, and many more. These can be produced by many kinds of meditation, certain exercise routines, the martial arts, hypnosis, psychoactive drugs, spiritual routines, and biofeedback among others.

Using the analogy from the last chapter, our minds are like computers, and our mindbody states are similar to programs. Like computer programs, each mindbody program accepts certain information, screens out other, transforms it, combines it with existing information, stores it, and uses it in various ways. Just as a person who has a computer can continually install new programs and learn to use them, humans can learn to use a variety of mindbody states. How many mindbody states are there? No one knows. Eastern psychologies such as Buddhism may have the best answer so far. But, whatever the number is, it is very large, probably in the hundreds, possibly in the thousands.

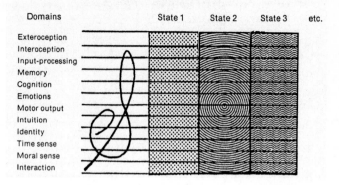

COMPOSITIONS FOR MIND
IN INFINITE VARIATIONS

Domains   State 1   State 2   State 3   etc.

Exteroception
Interoception
Input-processing
Memory
Cognition
Emotions
Motor output
Intuition
Identity
Time sense
Moral sense
Interaction

Another analogy I find useful as a way to think about the number of mindbody states is to compare each state/program to a musical composition for 12 'instruments', that is, for various combinations of 12 psychological processes. Just as each musical instrument can play a large number of notes, each mindbody process has many possible values.

These are from psychologist Charles Tart's 10 parameters or 'subsystems' of consciousness — read 'mindbody states.' Different combinations of these ingredients produce various mindbody states. Tart's 10 are: exteroception, interoception, input-processing, emotions, memory, time sense, sense of identity, evaluation and cognitive processing, motor output, and interaction with the environment.

I've added two more, making a dozen — 'moral sense' and 'intuition.' I added moral sense to recognize that moral judgments and values change when someone moves from a state that gives a sense of personal identity to a transpersonal state, one in which the sense of self evaporates. Here again my psychedelic-occasioned experiences of self-transcendence helped me understand the transpersonal shift and add its accompanying moral sense. I've added intuition to recognize this cognitive operator that acts as an inner guide.

It may be that this dozen instruments should be replaced by a different combo; in Chapter 11, we'll consider 11 parameters of consciousness that Benny Shanon proposes from his extensive study of the Brazilian psychoactive sacrament ayahuasca. One of the multistate topics where empirical and theoretical research most needs to be done is identifying the mental characteristics to pay attention to, the parameters, as they are called. It might turn out that different lists, different combos, may be useful for different purposes.

Describing and classifying these remains a task for future researchers. Eastern psychologies may have already done this for us; although, I expect Western mindsets will want to classify them differently. The most basic concept in this theory is *mindbody state,* and its full articulation remains a task for future mindbody explorers.

Mindbody Psychotechnologies

Mindbody psychotechnology is the second major concept in the multistate paradigm. Mindbody psychotechnologies are methods of producing various states. They include both traditional and new techniques such as meditation, yoga and other physical disciplines, psychoactive drugs, contemplative prayer and other spiritual practices, biofeedback, imagery and relaxation, sleep, hypnosis, the martial arts, and more. In the last several decades our culture has been importing traditional techniques from other cultures and developing new ones of our own.

William James's 1902 book *The Varieties of Religious Experience: A Study in Human Nature* started the mindbody ball rolling more than a century ago, but it was dropped during the Freudian era when all mindbody states other than our ordinary awake state were (incorrectly) seen as tainted by the unconscious. (That is, they were seen as at least a bit crazy). This singlestate error persisted during the Behaviorist era, when subjective experience was excluded from psychology, and such a word as 'mind' seemed unscientific, and 'mental' had an intellectually naughty odor to it.

Thanks to the clarion wake-up call from psychedelics in the 1960s and 70s, it became impossible to ignore other mindbody states and ways to achieve them. As a result, William James's paragraph about mindbody states in the epigraph to Chapter 8 became one of the most-quoted statements about the human mind, but the first two sentences with their reference to James's use of nitrous oxide were often omitted. Apparently, psychoactive drugs were also naughty enough to be deleted.

Although there were plenty of books about one or another mindbody state, it took Charles Tart's 1976 key book *Altered States of Consciousness* to make the point that psychoactive drugs, dreams, hypnosis, biofeedback, meditation, and so forth are all related to each other as part of the shared topic of altered states — 'mindbody studies' as I like to call them. Since 1976 books on specific states and books which recognized the combined mindbody field have been proliferating. Among my favorite multistate anthologies are Theodore X. Barber's *Advances in Altered States of Consciousness and Human Potentialities* and Michael Murphy's *The Future of the Body*.

A glance through the catalogs of online booksellers shows a large number of new books about psychedelics, and it may be my selective perception, but it seems to me the number is rising steadily. The popularization of 'new' psychoactive drugs such as DMT, ketamine, MDMA, and ayahuasca has certainly helped. In 2002 even the psychedelically stodgy American Psychological Association published *Varieties of Anomalous Experience*, whose chapter on mysticism includes the entheogenic uses of psychedelics, and in 2003 the APA published *Alterations of Consciousness*, which has a chapter on psychedelics.

Residency

'Residency' is the third major idea of multistate theory. 'Residency' is the idea that all human behavior and experience occur in mindbody states. That is, a mindbody state provides the psychophysiological context (program) from which all behavior and experience grow; alternately, one might say a mindbody state expresses or emits a behavior. Residency provides a useful assumption for two ways of exploring human capacities and for learning them. First, one can ask: 'In what state is this ability stronger or strongest? Can an ability be enhanced by performing it in a different mindbody state?' Second, 'Does each ability have analogs in other mindbody states? Are there different kinds or varieties of a specific ability in other mindbody states, say different kinds of intelligence, new cognitive skills, or different motivations?' In the Part 4, we'll look at implications for education. Meanwhile, Chapters 10 – 12 explore how these residency questions enrich our understanding of our minds.

Summary

I use ideas of *mindbody state*, *mindbody psychotechnology*, and *residency* to form the backbone of how I think about our multistate minds. Each lends itself to a working principle for guiding my thinking about what it means to have a mind and what it would mean to be fully educated:

Mindbody state: Humans produce and use a large number of mindbody states. Their number is not known. Existing states may be discovered in other cultures, and it may be possible to design and produce new ones.

Mindbody psychotechnology: There are many methods for producing mindbody states. New methods are being invented and imported into our culture.

Residency: Our mental and physical capacities exist, 'reside' within mindbody states. As we explore mindbody states, some abilities will strengthen and others weaken. Unknown, rare, and unusual abilities may reside in other mindbody states.

In addition to enriching how we can think about thinking (by paying attention to other states' thinking processes), these three ideas also challenge us to enter those states and think using their cognitive processes. In other words, the multistate view offers us both new things to think about and new thinking skills to think with. Additionally, psychedelics and other mindbody psychotechnologies make it possible to research subjective consciousness experimentally.

By spotting multistate contributions to intelligence and creative problem solving, the next chapter shows some practical advantages of a multistate paradigm. Then Chapter 11 will show how a multistate paradigm strengthens psychology as a science and other sciences too; that is, by compiling both psychedelic and nonpsychedelic psychotechnologies and by including more complete information about our minds, a multistate perspective gives us a fuller view of our capacities, behavior, and experience. Access to a variety of mindbody states may even contribute to the competitive survival of people who have multistate skills over those whose limits are restricted by singlestate minds. At the very least, used wisely, they can improve our daily lives.

Chapter 10

Intelligence, Creativity, Metaintelligence

To start out, it's helpful to notice that our current definitions of intelligence all have to do with optimally using our usual awake state, and we call someone intelligent (We should probably say 'singlestate intelligent.') if he or she uses this state well. Multistate theory invites us to extend our ideas of intelligence to other states. Demonstrating this extension, two widely used theories of intelligence show the limits of singlestate IQ theory and at the same time provide launching pads for multistate extensions. These are the theories of Howard Gardner and Robert Sternberg.

Increasing Intelligence — Creative Problem Solving

Cognitive psychologist Howard Gardner, a professor at Harvard, is best known for his theory of Multiple Intelligences. He defines intelligence as the ability to solve problems or produce goods and services of value in a society. However, Gardner, like most specialists in intelligence, limits his examples of intelligences to our ordinary awake state, but people have used other mindbody states to help solve problems in the past. Dreams provide many examples. For example, author Robert Louis Stevenson dreamed some of his plots. French philosopher Condorcet solved a difficult mathematical equation in his sleep. Poet William Blake dreamed that his dead brother instructed him in an engraving technique. Kekule literally dreamed up the benzene ring; and archeologist Hilprecht dreamed about a priest of Nipper who showed him how to decipher Babylonian cuneiform characters by fitting together artifacts that previously had seemed unrelated to each other. Since they solved problems during dreams, don't these indicate dream-state intelligence?

> The second thing I would like to discuss is the increase in intuition that occurs in the psychedelic experience — sometimes a frightening increase. ... There's a tremendous increase in ... being able to look at something as it is now and see in it those immanent forces which will make it something different in the future — and also in perceiving what that future might be. There's a sort of cutting through conventional posture — including one's own.
>
> Frank Barron
> *The Creative Process and
> the Psychedelic Experience*

Problem solving (Gardner's foundation concept in his definition of intelligence) also exists during psychedelic states and may be enhanced by them. The best known study is 'Psychedelic Agents in Creative Problem Solving: A Pilot Study,' published in *Psychological Reports* in 1966. After they screened and prepared their subjects, Willis Harman, a Professor of Engineering Economic Systems at Stanford, and his collaborators gave LSD to 27 men in groups of 3 or 4. They were 'engaged in various professional occupations, i.e., engineers, physicists, mathematicians, architects, a furniture designer, and a commercial artist and had a total of 44 professional problems they wanted to work on.' They all were stumped by problems they had been previously working on but without success.

During the sessions, they relaxed and listened to music during a 'quiet period.' Later, after snacks and informally discussing their problem with the others in their small groups, they each spent 3 to 4 hours working by themselves on their respective problems.

Harman's 27 problem-solvers typically described the following subjective results among others:

- Capacity to structure problems in a larger context.
- High fluency and flexibility of ideation.
- High capacity for visual imagery.
- High ability to concentrate.
- Accessibility of unconscious resources.
- Ability to associate seemingly dissimilar elements in meaningful ways.
- Capacity to visualize the completed solution in its entirety.

These cognitive processes form part of the backbone of creativity, and the practical results were impressive. Insights into academic problems included a mathematical theorem and a new conceptual model of a photon. They solved engineering problems, including one on space-probes, another on an electron accelerator beam-steering device, and improvements to a magnetic tape recorder. Design problems solved included a chair, furniture line, and a letterhead. The architects envisioned projects that were accepted by clients, including a commercial building and a private dwelling. These psychedelic creativity sessions certainly meet Gardner's criterion for intelligence as the ability to solve problems of value to a society.

If intelligence includes using dreams and/or psychedelic states to produce products and services of value in a culture, can people become more intelligent by learning to access dream-based thinking and psychedelic-based thinking and learning to use their respective cognitive processes? Can we learn to increase dream intelligence? How? And dreams are just one mindbody example. Hypnosis, meditation, and other mindbody states may house their respective kinds of intelligence too. When we learn to use our minds' many mindbody mental 'programs', will this boost our creative problem solving? Will we discover new reservoirs of intelligence? What unknown cognitive skills might we discover and develop when we learn to use our minds in new ways? These questions excite prospectors of the multistate mind to look at other states too. The next chapter follows these indications further.

Increasing Intelligence — Learning New Cognitive Processes

A particularly interesting instance of psychedelic-assisted problem solving comes from Nobel Prize winner Kary Mullis, and it exemplifies a different kind of multistate intelligence when he invented the PCR technique. What is PCR? When trying to do research on biological specimens, sometimes the sample is too small to use. Mullis solved the small-sample problem by inventing the PCR technique. PCR (polymerase chain reaction) allows biologists to increase the size of, say, a DNA sample so that the specimen is large enough for scientists to do research on it.

> There are a lot of people for whom psychedelics have been really beneficial. But I wouldn't recommend it to everyone. Some people are just not ready but society would benefit from letting people who are ready for psychedelics have legal access to them.
>
> Kary Mullis

Thus, Mullis' invention made it possible to advance lines of research that had been stalled before his invention.

In terms of mindbody theory, the intriguing thing about Mullis' insight was not that it occurred during an LSD session. It didn't. Instead, Mullis learned a visual thinking skill during LSD sessions and transferred that visualization skill back to his ordinary state to solve the small-sample problem.

An even better known insight into biology, and another Nobel winning one too, is Francis Crick's double helix model of DNA, and that had its birth thanks to LSD too. Among the laudatory obituaries when Crick died in 2004 was 'Nobel Prize genius Crick was high on LSD when he discovered the secret of life.' In the article, which appeared in the London newspaper *Mail on Sunday*, journalist Alun Rees reported, '[Crick] said it was LSD, not the Eagle's [a pub] warm beer, that helped him to unravel the structure of DNA, the discovery that won him the Nobel Prize.'

When he interviewed Richard Kemp, who as young biochemist in the 70's knew Crick and who later 'devised the world's first foolproof method of producing cheap, pure LSD,' Rees uncovered what may be a clue to higher power thinking that has not-yet been followed up, but that deserves further investigation both for the history of ideas and as a clue to upgrading cognitive skills and raising fertile ideas:

> Dick Kemp told me he met Francis Crick at Cambridge. Crick had told him that some Cambridge academics used LSD in tiny amounts as a thinking tool, to liberate them from preconceptions and let their genius wander freely to new ideas. Crick told him he had perceived the double-helix shape while on LSD. (Rees, 2004)

The biological sciences and medicine have benefited from psychedelics in a more general way too. Psychedelics piqued the minds of many young scientists and boosted their curiosity about the biochemistry of our nervous system and our personal experiences. How could such a tiny amount of a chemical cause such immense changes in how we feel, think, and perceive? What is going on in our brains? Discovering that LSD has a similar chemical structure to the neurotransmitter serotonin energized novelty seeking scientists to explore the similarities, some with microscopes in their laboratories, others with headphones in their living rooms, some with both.

Within the neurosciences, this connection is a widely acknowledged 'secret.'

At the 1999 Annual Meeting of the Society for Neuroscience, Dr. David E. Nichols, Professor in the Department of Medicinal Chemistry and Molecular Pharmacology at Purdue University, brought this scientific secret out of the psychedelic closet. Whether their interest came from their own psychedelic experiences, because they noted the structural similarity between the serotonin molecule and psychedelics' structure, perhaps from wondering what people enjoy about these experiences, or from the perspective of psychotherapy or even drug law enforcement, Dave Nichols observed, 'Whatever the motivation, I would still assert that a significant percentage of the serotonin researchers in the world today developed their research focus through some connection to psychedelic drugs.'

As Nichols said, in a very real sense, psychedelics jump started the neurosciences and greatly increased the flow of ideas from the biological tributary into the river of cognitive studies. In the table on page 127, 'A Comparison of Singlestate and Multistate Paradigms — Cognition' the distinctions between singlestate and multistate paradigms come from recognizing that we can use our minds in many mindbody states. Psychedelics are by no means the only source of these ideas, but they are one major source. Why did these ideas appear when they did and where they did? Knowledge about meditation, contemplative prayer, psychoactive plants, the martial arts, sensory deprivation, and similar mindbody psychotechnologies has been around for thousands of years. Why have these practices and the ideas they elicit suddenly become so acceptable since the 1960s? Psychedelics.

They're both Electric — Chemicals and Computers

Biotechnology isn't the only technology with psychedelic genes. Electronics and computers share psychedelic chromosomes too. Shareware owes its life to psychedelic experiences, and its invention is another instance of a cognitive skill learned in a psychedelic mindbody state, then transferred back to our ordinary state. In 'Psychedelic Science,' one of the BBC-TV's *Horizon* series, Bob Wallace described his novel solution to a common business problem of product distribution this way:

> The big quandary for software companies was getting into the market place, finding shelf space. But there was a new way of doing that I thought of called 'shareware,' and I think the concept was very unusual, and I think the concept came to some extent from my psychedelic experience. In shareware you give away the software, and then you encourage people to pay for it, and even though a low percentage of people might pay for it, so many people use it that the percentage of return back is really pretty good. So that worked. That worked pretty well. (*Horizon: Psychedelic Science*)

Was shareware just another silly, stoned idea? Did it help the company that used it? Both the shareware business strategy and the company that used it are beneficiaries of psychedelic based intelligence — shareware and Microsoft. Micrograms for Microsoft.

A Comparison of Singlestate and Multistate Paradigms

— Cognition —

(MBS = mindbody state)

ASSUMPTIONS OF SINGLESTATE PSYCHOLOGIES	ASSUMPTIONS OF MULTISTATE PSYCHOLOGIES
Cognition	
Cognition during MBSs other than our usual MBS is inferior.	Different MBSs are major shifts of cognitive processing. Some may contain useful styles of thinking. A complete cognitive psychology would include them.
Advanced Cognition	
Secondary process thinking is adult, rational thinking and is done in an awake state. All other forms of thinking are irrational, childlike, and useless.	Advanced cognition (tertiary process thinking) includes the selection of an appropriate MBS or sequence of MBSs for the task at hand.
Cognitive Development	
Abstract, formal, adult reasoning is the highest level of cognitive development.	Selecting and using one's MBSs is a higher level of cognitive development.
Reduction/Emergence	
Thoughts, values, and beliefs are the result of underlying biological processes.	Thoughts, values, beliefs and other conscious or mental phenomena exert emergent or downward causation on human behavior, biology, & experience.
Intelligence	
Intelligence is the ability to use our awake state skillfully.	Intelligence is the ability to use every mindbody state skillfully and the metaintelligence to select the appropriate MBSs for desired goals.
Creativity and Problem Solving	
Linear, rational, sequential thought is the best way to solve scientific and personal problems.	Many insightful and valuable ideas occur during non-ordinary states.

The Multistate Cognitive Horizon

When we broaden the horizon of intelligence to include multistate intelligence, an obvious parallel is that we're also looking at a wider horizon for all cognition. The table above contrasts a singlestate view of cognition with a multistate view. And it's worth reminding ourselves that the traits being compared are generalizations and may not hold in every case.

We shouldn't neglect the dot-mil people. When the US Navy was working on a difficult problem in pattern recognition in its intelligence equipment, one of its researchers sailed off on an LSD trip and solved the problem: 'With LSD,' said a retired Navy Captain, 'the normal limiting mechanisms of the brain are released, and entirely new patterns of perception emerge.'

Similarly, are there other cognitive skills residing in other mindbody states that we can learn in those states? Can we use them in those states — as in the examples from dreams and Harman's creative problem solving? Or can we transfer them back into our ordinary state — as in the case of Mullis? Can we increase the number and kinds of cognitive skills at our command? A multistate perspective answers 'yes.'

This increased diversity in thinking skills brings up the way another cognitive psychologist defines 'intelligence.' Former Yale cognitive psychologist Robert Sternberg — now Dean of Arts and Sciences at Tufts — defines intelligence as 'mental self-management;' although, he too applies his definition only to our ordinary awake state. If we extend his definition to other mental programs (states), it is logical that someone who can access and use a larger repertoire of mindbody programs has more mental self-management options and flexibility (is more intelligent) than someone with a more limited selection (someone like most of us most of the time). Mullis shows this second kind of multistate intelligence. He increased his mental self-management by learning a new cognitive skill. Extending Sternberg's ideas about intelligence to include multistate thinking suggests that parallel opportunities for practical problem solving, scholarly thinking, intellectual invention, scientific ideas, and artistic possibilities may flourish when we escape the constrictions of the singlestate fallacy.

So we have two ways of boosting intelligence here. The first — Harman's LSD research and Crick's DNA insight — provides solutions to specific problems during psychedelic sessions. In this it resembles problem solving in dreams. It teaches us that we can solve problems in other mindbody states that we can't (or don't) solve in our ordinary, awake state. The second — Mullis' PCR insight and Wallace's shareware idea — teaches us that we can develop new cognitive skills during other mindbody states and transfer them back to our ordinary state to use there afterwards.

The ability to learn new cognitive skills in different mindbody states raises a swarm of questions: Are there other useful cognitive skills residing in other mindbody states? What are they? Which states do they reside in? How do we gain access to the states and learn these skills? What would it mean for humanity to have new ways to increase intelligence or add new cognitive skills to our mental repertoire? No matter how psychologists define 'intelligence' or 'cognition,' it is time to extend these definitions to include different kinds of thinking lying undiscovered and underdeveloped in mindbody states other than our ordinary awake state.

Metaintelligence

What about someone who is highly skilled at selecting mindbody states, achieving them, and using their resident abilities? Presumably, this more general ability leads to creativity, solving problems, producing useful goods, and advances in thinking. It seems to me that achieving and using various mindbody states (including their cognitive programs) are kinds of metaintelligence. This background or executive intelligence is the ability to select the best cognitive program for our purpose at the time. Multistate metaintelligence would also help us discover and develop other more state–specific intelligences.

Since intelligence and problem solving strengthen in some states (and weaken in others) do our other psychological processes vary too? This question opens the door to what, to me at least, looks like 'the major intellectual opportunity of our times', and we'll get to that in the chapter after next in our mental hike through psychedelia. But in order to more fully appreciate the impact of that major intellectual opportunity, first it's helpful to widen our perspective beyond this chapter's focus on intelligence and problem solving, so in Chapter 11 we'll look at psychology, science, and survival by locating them along our multistate horizons.

[T]he bringing together of Ayahuasca research and cognitive psychology defines a two-way interaction. Not only can a cognitive-psychological analysis make a crucial contribution to the study of Ayahuasca, the converse is also the case — the study of Ayahuasca may have implications of import to our general understanding of the workings of the human mind. Ayahuasca (along with other mind-altering substances) expands the horizons of psychology and reveals new, hitherto unknown territories of the mind. Thus, the study of Ayahuasca presents new data pertaining to human consciousness, and thus new issues for investigation, new ways to look at things, new questions, and perhaps even new answers.

Benny Shanon
The Antipodes of the Mind (p. 37)

Chapter 11

Psychology, Science, and Survival

As we saw in Chapter 9, some ideas are so fundamental to what we think that when they change they set off a domino cascade in the line of ideas downstream from them. Our view of our minds is a top-domino idea. In this chapter we'll sample downstream ideas in psychology, scientific standards, and human survival. Our little idea-snacks are by no means the full multistate menu, but they'll give us a taste of ideas yet to come.

In psychology we'll consider psychedelics as a way to explore the cognitive unconscious, what to pay attention to when we look into our minds (its parameters).

In the sciences we'll look toward broader databases that include observations from all mindbody states and theory that includes them. This will lead us to a multistate criterion for judging scientific generalizations and to a multistate way to design interdisciplinary studies.

Our prehistoric ancestors advanced when they learned to make the hand axe and discovered agriculture. Our generations are steadily advancing our use of computer-based information technology toward its fullest capacity. Similarly, as we learn to increase our repertoire of mindbody psychotechnologies, will we advance the ways we use our brains and minds? By the end of this chapter, we'll be looking at the multistate mind as an adaptive advantage for individuals, groups, and our species.

Psychology

Psychology, psychedelics and other mindbody methods give us new topics to think about such as other states and the cognitive, emotional, and bodily processes that may reside in them. For example: How many states are there? How do we achieve them? What skills do they contain? Those are some of the questions we'll introduce in this chapter, and this chapter will pave the way for Chapters 12–14, which will elaborate this approach and some of its uses in education.

In addition to providing mindbody states as processes to study, a second advantage gives us new mental skills to think with — original ways to use our minds, new thinking processes, new cognitive skills. When we discover and develop new cognitive skills in other mindbody states, we have done more than map a new part of our minds. We now have the advantage of using those processes to think with. Questions about which ones will be useful for what purposes are another direction for researchers to explore. In this chapter, we'll look at some of these advantages. Our discussion in this chapter will warm us up to consider the Central Multistate Question in Chapter 12.

The sciences which study our minds are the direct beneficiaries of a third set of advantages. We'll look into ways of studying our minds in greater detail, identifying neglected psychological parameters, solving problems and creativity, raising intelligence, including novel ideas about our minds, establishing multistate criteria for judging scientific generalizations, asking new questions, and spotting multistate-based opportunities for interdisciplinary research.

The Cognitive Unconscious — Viewing the Floors of Conception

One of psychedelics' psychomagnifying benefits is casting light on parts of our minds that are usually out of sight. For psychologists who are interested in repressed memories and fantasies, psychedelics can bring them to awareness. For those interested in the possibility of birth memories, even these can be re-experienced thanks to the psychedelics' psychomagnifying power. Jungians can use psychedelics to access the collective unconscious, including archetypes. And cognitive psychologists can amplify the ideas and assumptions that lurk below our usual threshold of awareness. All of these affect what we do, think, and feel. In fact, to a great extent they determine are sense of who we are.

'Know Thyself' is one of the 3 precepts carved into the temple of the oracle in ancient Delphi, and psychedelics aid us in knowing ourselves too. First, by carrying our awareness down into our minds, they let us see the lower floors of conception, the deep layers from which our thoughts and feelings arise. For example, anthropologist of consciousness Michael Winkelman calls psychedelics 'psychointegrators.' As senior lecturer in the Department of Anthropology at Arizona State University and Director of the Ethnographic Field School in Ensenada, Mexico, for 15 years, Winkelman's interest in consciousness lead him to become a founding member of the Society for the Anthropology of Consciousness.

By integrating neural, sensory, and cognitive processes, psychointegrators (psychedelics) allow 'the enhancement of access to deeper cognitive structures.' In an article in the summer 2002 issue of *ENTHEOS: The Journal of Psychedelic Spirituality*, he summarizes:

> ... The paleomammalian brain manages processes associated with self, identity, species survival, family and social relations, learning and memory, and sexual

and aggressive emotions as well as their behavior integration. Entheogens [psychedelics] (and ASC in general) enhance systematic integration of the psyche by producing heightened [magnified] arousal and awareness, and by interfering with habituated behavioral routines. The paleomammalian brain and limbic system provide the social and emotional mentation and behavior. These fundamental cognitive processes involve nonverbal communication, and forms of mental and social representation that manage the processes of emotional and social life. (pp. 56–7)

In other words, psychedelics strengthen the communication between the lower parts of our brains that give us our sense of personal identity, attachment and social bonding, emotion, conviction (in beliefs); and the higher neocortex, where our higher level thinking takes place. Increased communication also goes laterally as communication between brain hemispheres also increases. Presumably, increasing the inside-the-brain communication produces psychotherapeutic effects.

At other times it gives a sense of primary religious experience, of 'The Divine Other.' The interplay between entheogens and religion is one of my major interests, but is beyond the scope of this book.

A cautionary reminder is due at this point. Not all psychedelic sessions will always do these things. Like any other psychedelic experience, these experiences are 'sometime things.' And psychedelic explorers have to be willing and able to face frightening memories, imagined fears, undesirable ideas, and terrifying emotions for these sometimes lurk in the basements of our minds too.

When information flows from the lower floors of our minds up to the higher floors, we become aware of what's going on downcellar. By helping us explore these hidden floors of conception that we usually aren't aware of, psychedelics give us a new and deeper relationship with our minds. They provide a method to follow the Delphic precept 'Know Thyself.'

Hunting Our Minds' Wild Parameters

Psychedelics also benefit the humanities, sciences, and especially cognitive studies by pointing out important characteristics of our minds that we might otherwise miss. Until recently, most people paid attention primarily to how psychedelics magnified emotions, enlarged emotionally-laden ideas, or influenced the senses. In 2002 this changed when Oxford University Press published *The Antipodes of the Mind*; a cognitive direction opened in psychedelic studies. *Antipodes* is a book about the cognitive implications of the Brazilian psychoactive sacrament ayahuasca, and its author, Benny Shanon, is well respected within the cognitive sciences.

Shanon addressed an unresolved problem with thinking about different mindbody states (a.k.a. states of consciousness, psychophysiological states, mindbody programs). As we move through these states, what kinds of things should we pay attention to? It's easy to get so absorbed by the specific thoughts, experiences, and the oddities we see, or by the intense feelings that we fail to notice cognitive events such as thinking, perceiving, sense of self, and changes in rational processes. Broader characteristics that mind explorers should take note of often get lost. Important things that change are called 'parameters.' As a sort of check list of what changes, they remind us what to pay attention to so that we'll have a complete account of each state. In altered-state explorations, they remind us to pay attention not only to the fascinating experiences we have but also to the broader mindbody parameters that vary from state to state.

What parameters do we become aware of when we use psychedelics or other mindbody techniques? The author of *Antipodes*, Benny Shanon, is a professor of psychology at Hebrew University in Jerusalem. He has served as a visiting professor internationally, including visiting professorships in France, England, the US, Poland, Italy, Brazil, and the Netherlands. In addition to having over 100 articles published and presenting over 150 papers at meetings, he has served on committees that referee submitted papers for over 2 dozen professional journals.

The Antipodes of the Mind: Charting the Phenomenology of the Ayahuasca Experience illustrates the value of psychedelics (and by implication other mindbody psychotechnologies) as methods of exploring our minds. They alert us to parameters that we might otherwise miss. Shanon's chapter 'Consciousness I' sketches this task:

> Thus from a structural point of view, consciousness can be defined as the set of parameters that specify the particular way human beings experience the world, both physical and mental. (p. 195)

> The great potential contribution of the study of non-ordinary states of consciousness to the scientific understanding of the mind lies precisely in their rendering the parameters of the cognitive system apparent and in their revealing the various possible values that these parameters may take. (p. 196)

Informing his investigations of ayahuasca with his years as a cognitive psychologist, Shanon identifies 11 structural parameters of consciousness and some of the unusual values they can take:

- Agenthood — experiencing thoughts as not being one's own
- Personal identity — personal identification with whatever one is looking at, a sense of unity with the other
- Unity — being oneself at the same time being someone or something else

- Boundaries — erasing the boundary between inner and outer reality
- Individuation — self transcendence but with consciousness still maintained
- Calibration — change in perceptions of one's size, weight, posture, etc.
- Locus of consciousness — consciousness located outside one's physical body
- Time — variations in time, including its speed or even feelings of eternity
- Self-consciousness — a 'residue' of the normal self after other facets of consciousness are completely altered
- Intentionality — no object to which thought is being directed and no content entertained by the mind, often leading to a sense of 'the Void' or 'pure consciousness.'
- Connectedness, Knowledge, and the Conferral of Reality — a powerful sense of knowing, a noetic sense.

He describes these in much greater detail in his book. This list reminds other consciousness researchers about what to pay attention to when they describe non-ordinary experiences, say, during different types of meditation, when they construct surveys of people who practice various martial arts, or develop interview protocols about mindbody experiences. Because Shanon is a cognitive psychologist, the parameters he selected reflect cognitive interests. People with other interests would choose to pay attention to other parameters. For example, Stan Grof exemplifies more interest in emotions. Working originally with a group of mental patients in clinical settings, psychiatrist Stan Grof organized his patients' experiences by the depth of mind they seemed to come from: abstract and

A Comparison of Singlestate and Multistate Paradigms

— Psychologies —

MBS = mindbody state

ASSUMPTIONS OF SINGLESTATE PSYCHOLOGIES	ASSUMPTIONS OF MULTISTATE PSYCHOLOGIES
Psychology	
Psychology is the study of behavior and experiences (primarily in our usual MBS).	A complete psychology must include all MBSs. Which psychological principles apply only to our ordinary MBS, and which apply across several states?
State of Consciousness	
MBS depends on the physical, biological, chemical, and electrical state of the brain and body.	The physical, biological, chemical, and electrical states of the brain and body can be voluntarily controlled to an unknown extent; therefore, MBS is a controllable variable.
Freudian	
The unconscious is a repository of repressed experiences and fantasies. Psychotherapy occurs when these contents are made conscious, i.e., put under the control of the ego.	Freud did not recognize development beyond the ego. Mental and physical healing are often associated with access to selected MBSs.
Behaviorism	
In the SORC model (stimulus → organism → response → consequence) the O can be omitted because it is a constant for all practical purposes.	The biological state of the organism (the O) is a significant variable from MBS to MBS. Stimuli, responses, and reinforcements also vary from MBS to MBS.
Humanistic Psychology and Self-Actualization	
Self-actualization is the top of Maslow's needs hierarchy.	Self-transcendence is a stage beyond self-actualization in Maslow's needs hierarchy.

Continued on next page

Continued from previous page

ASSUMPTIONS OF SINGLESTATE PSYCHOLOGIES	ASSUMPTIONS OF MULTISTATE PSYCHOLOGIES
Transpersonal	
The standard unit of analysis in psychology is the separate, individual person and/or the actions of collectivities of separate individuals.	MBSs may be divided into those that produce a sense of separate, individual being (personal MBSs) and those which give a sense of unified wholeness (transpersonal MBSs).
Social Psychology	
Social psychology studies the Interactions between individual persons and/or the actions of collections of collections of individuals.	The perception of personal separateness is a function of our ordinary MBS. Social relationships vary from MBS to MBS.
Positive Psychology	
Flow, satisfaction, and positive feelings, as well as almost all other desirable human characteristics occur in our normal MBS.	A full understanding of positive psychology would acknowledge that peak performance, creative insight, and subjectively beneficial emotions often occur in extraordinary MBSs.

aesthetic, personal biographies, the perinatal (birth) level, and the transpersonal level.

It's important to notice that one of psychedelic's benefits is to call our attention to what to pay attention to: What are the important parameters of our minds? Because psychedelics can change our experience so much, they help us with this question. Parameters that we might otherwise overlook in a singlestate view are now in plain view, such as the noetic sense and self-transcendence. As people explore other states, we can expect more significant parameters to emerge. One multistate step at a time, the unresolved issue of what is best to pay attention to will be elaborated.

Science

Another benefit from the multistate approach is a stronger more complete science, one that includes the full range of data. As these chapters show, the scientific endeavor expands from investigating one state to investigating many, from using the thinking of skills of one state to using those of many. The first increases what multistate scientists explore, the second increases the cognitive processes they can use.

Until the recent decades, our current, singlestate paradigm ignored observations about human behavior, experience, and skills which occur in states other than our normal awake state. This has been slowly changing as science expands to consider such things as meditation, dreams, psychopharmacology, and the biological correlates of various altered states. However, these fields too often see themselves as unconnected with each other, thus one contribution of a multistate view is encouraging them to see themselves as part of a developing, leading edge, multistate frontier of science and a still larger field of multistate studies.

Broader Databases

Even when we take the recent advances in these growing fields into account, the sciences that study the human mind are still heavily anchored in singlestate research. Consequently our knowledge about our minds and their processes displays a sampling error; we selectively draw our data from only our ordinary, awake mindbody state. With its emphasis on understanding the full range of human experience, the multistate paradigm accepts information about all mindbody states as necessary to our understanding of human nature. As philosopher Alfred North Whitehead said, '... the rejection of any source of evidence is always treason to that ultimate rationalism which urges forward science and philosophy alike' (p. vii).

If we are to have the fullest understanding of human nature, then we must include the evidence about all mindbody states, not just one. The multistate paradigm promises us a richer, more complete sample of human behavior and experience.

> The most important obligation of any science is that its descriptive and theoretical language embrace *all* the phenomena of its subject matter; the data from [altered states of consciousness] cannot be ignored if we are to have a comprehensive psychology.
>
> Charles T. Tart
> *Altered States of Consciousness* (p. 5)

Evaluating Generalizations and Theories — The Criterion of Multistate Breadth

In addition to providing a broader framework for considering more data and asking new questions, the multistate paradigm gives us a new standard for judging scientific claims about our minds. Because scientists hope to find principles that apply to many situations, a common rule for evaluating a generalization's strength is: the wider the range of observations, the stronger the conclusion. Other things being equal, findings based on observations from several mindbody states are stronger than those derived from one state, so based on this criterion, most current generalizations in psychology, the social sciences, and education will be strengthened if they are informed by observations from several states. Testing our current singlestate knowledge in other states is a major opportunity for generations of researchers.

Toward Integrated Mindbody Studies

The multistate paradigm's power is not just that it requires us to include information about all states when we think about our minds. It does this. But more than this, it provides a structure for integrating and organizing topics which have been — and still are — a disconnected collection of miscellaneous specialties. As things now stand, hypnosis, dreaming, psychoactive drugs, meditation, and so forth are separate strands of research. Each mindbody specialty proceeds along its own road only occasionally contacting the other specialties. By reassembling specific, separate strands, multistate studies encourages cross fertilization of findings and communication among disciplines.

For example: How do various kinds of meditation and psychedelics interact? Two works by Myron Stolaroff illustrate how meditation and psychedelics might mutually benefit each other. Stolaroff retired as Assistant to the President of Ampex Corporation in charge of long-range planning, where he contributed to Ampex's invention of the video tape recorder. Ampex is one of the grandparent companies of today's Silicon Valley high technology companies. In 1961 Stolaroff left Ampex to found the International Foundation for Advanced Study. There for 3½ years, and after careful screening and preparation, people could legally have carefully guided LSD experiences. In his book *Thanatos to Eros*, Stolaroff suggests that meditation practice would be good readiness training for psychedelic experiences. Making connections to another mindbody psychotechnology, he suggests: when it is legally possible to do so, preliminary MDMA sessions may be good training-wheel experiences to help people become used to altered states. And after acclimatizing people with easy first mindbody steps, MDMA could provide an emotionally positive first-stage liftoff for stronger psychedelic launchings. Stolaroff's interest in combining meditation, psychedelics, and MDMA illustrates a next step in mindbody thought, investigating the interactions among mindbody psychotechnologies.

The psychedelics-meditation influence may run in the other direction too. In his article 'Are Psychedelics Useful in the Practice of Buddhism?,' which appeared in the *Journal of Humanistic Psychology* in 1999, Stolaroff answers his question 'yes' with some qualifications: 'I personally have found that appropriately understood and used, psychedelics can play a significant role in deepening and accelerating the progress of one's meditative practice.'

A cluster of studies relates psychedelics to meditation, especially to Tibetan Buddhism. These are interesting themselves, especially to people who are interested in religion and the psychology of religion. From a mindbody perspective, these scholarly writings and empirical studies are a guiding light for interfacing two or more mindbody psychotechnologies. In 'Influences of Previous Psychedelic Drug Experiences on Students of Tibetan Buddhism' Charles Tart asked participants at a Buddhist 10-day retreat to fill out a questionnaire about their drug use. Ninety-four percent reported previous experience with marijuana and 77% experience with a major psychedelic. When rating how important psychedelics were to their general spiritual development, 52% said they were *very* or *fairly* important. Here a multistate view connects psychopharmacology and religion.

Stolaroff's and Tart's findings echo psychiatrist Roger Walsh's in-depth personal interviews from his chapter 'Psychedelics and Self-Actualization' in Grinspoon and Bakalar's *Psychedelic Reflections*. The chapter adds a study of mental health to the psychopharmacology-and-religion stew. While researching self-actualization, Walsh interviewed in depth 5 'of the healthiest Westerners who fit Maslow's criteria for self-actualization.' In order to establish that they weren't dropouts or irresponsible, Walsh

selected them because, they had eminent national or international reputations in their fields, had published at least
one book. Four were successful as teachers of psychology,
a mindbody discipline, or meditation. As he got to know
these 5 spiritual leaders and established their trust, he
found that their psychedelic experiences led them to recognize experiences, modes of self, and states of consciousness beyond our day-to-day experience. They reported a
new interest in depth psychology, religion, spirituality,
and consciousness, and related disciplines such as meditation. They mentioned intense emotions such as love, compassion, or empathy, and the recognition that the mind
can be and should be trained. Their psychedelic experiences sometimes supplied a guiding direction and meaning for their lives. Chapter 13's epigraph comes from this
study.

Clearly, Walsh is not saying that these 5 people typify
all users of psychedelics or that psychedelics are an
automatic step toward professional eminence. Just as
clearly, psychedelics can be misused. However, his point
is clear: psychedelics do open one path toward exploring
the mindbody universe, a path these self-actualizers followed. However, as Walsh reported: 'They took it as
self-evident that there are many people who should not
take psychedelics, especially anyone with significant psychological disturbances. However, they agreed that used
skillfully by a mature person, they could be helpful.'

Here again, psychedelics provide another instance of
how mindbody psychotechnologies can weave together
previously separate strands of interest — here psychopharmacology, psychology, cognition, religion, and ethics.
More than merely spotting relations among disciplines,
mindbody techniques provide ways to experiment
between these topics. Because mindbody states encompass things from chemicals and nerve firing to beliefs and
social context, mindbody studies provides natural con-

duits for interdisciplinary research. When researchers change something at one level (an independent variable) — such as a psychoactive drug — and look for changes at another level (a dependent variable) — such as religious and philosophical beliefs — they are truly doing cross-disciplinary research. For example, they can change the context where a mindbody psychotechnology is used and look for bodily changes or alterations in cognitions. In the next chapter we'll pick up on this theme in the section 'Consilience.'

In my judgment, scholars who fail to ask mindbody questions are restricting their own findings, failing in their intellectual responsibilities, and confining their disciplines.

Survival — Adaptive Advantage

Do 'increased mental flexibility,' 'more behavioral options,' and 'a variety of responses' sound familiar? Biologists recognize these traits as leading to species' adaptability and survival. To anthropologists they nourish flourishing cultures. Whether one thinks of evolution in the usual way as movement from the simple to the complex or as the spread of excellence via increased variation, learning other states' thinking skills makes us more cognitively complex and boosts human adaptability with a wider variety of mental and physical skills.

It seems credible to me that a nation which develops a fuller repertoire of its citizens' mental abilities will prosper more than one which develops fewer ways of thinking. The same principle applies to companies and their employees and universities and their professors. Besides mentioning Harman's problem solving sessions, a BBC TV documentary *Psychedelic Science* reported the often rumored and widely believed story that many of the advances in computer design and engineering were solved during psychedelic and/or marijuana states. It may be no accident that Silicon Valley mines the rich mindbody vein running through the San Francisco Bay Area.

The competitive multistate advantage should be especially strong over nations and organizations that anchor themselves in singlestate thinking, neglecting other states, marginalizing them, or even outlawing the mindbody psychotechnologies which produce them. If we increase the repertoire of cognitive programs we use, will this help us develop increasingly complex thinking and sophisticated problem solving? Will a multistate project advance humanity more steps along our long-term cognitive evolution?

Summary

Psychedelics lead to new ways to explore our minds. They help us plumb our mind's cognitive and emotional depths. By displaying different ways our minds can operate, they remind us of previously neglected parameters. By invigorating new thinking processes, they strengthen intelligence and boost creative problem solving. They point to new kinds of intelligence in other mindbody states. Opening the door to a multistate view, psychedelics critique our current knowledge as systematically excluding information about other states, and they remind us to check whether our generalizations about the human mind are limited to information from only our ordinary, awake state. Psychedelics and other mindbody methods provide ways to do interdisciplinary research. Improved skills and new tools contribute to survival. Will psychedelics and other mindbody skills strengthen this process?

I expect one of the most productive areas for ideas and inventions will be future generations of information technologies, biotechnologies, and psychotechnologies, especially their children who will hybridize genes from all three parents. In my own thinking, I'm not clear about whether spiritual technologies are a child of these three parents or a fourth, separate genetic line, perhaps some of both

Where do we go from here? This question is a clue: How does intelligence vary from mindbody state to mindbody state? This is one example of what I call the 'Central Multistate Question'. And we can ask parallel questions of many scholarly, scientific, educational, and psychological topics. In the next chapter the box 'The Central Multistate Question' illustrates the fruitfulness of this question-germinating approach. The same approach applies to education. All the standard questions of education — What can be known? What thinking skills are there? How do we teach them? — these and other questions get reasked. In Chapter 13, the matrix 'All the Questions Get Reasked' outlines this blueprint for education.

Chapter 12

The Major Intellectual Opportunity of Our Times –

The Central Multistate Question

Besides promoting broader databases and a criterion for judging generalizations, the multistate paradigm offers a broader philosophical critique of our current methods of knowing. We use our minds to study reality. What are the limits to knowledge in our ordinary state? When we learn to use our minds in new ways (in new mindbody states), what will we discover about reality?

Our minds are also the primary instruments we use in all our knowing. They are capable of perceiving, thinking, intuiting, et cetera in many mindbody states, yet we use them in only one of their modes. This makes almost everything we know an artifact constructed by our minds' ordinary awake program

I'm not claiming that everything we know is wrong or that observations and ideas in altered states are any more accurate than those in our ordinary state. In fact, assuming that our ordinary state has evolved during millennia as our mental home base, I suppose this state has survival value. I suppose it is the most functional state, but that doesn't mean it's the only useful state or that other states have no uses.

As psychiatrist Kubie pointed out in another context:

> A discipline comes of age and a student of that discipline reaches maturity when it becomes possible to recognize, estimate and allow for the errors of their tools. ... Yet there is one instrument which every discipline uses without checking its errors. This, of course, is the human psychological apparatus. (p. 349)

While Kubie was discussing the influence of the unconscious, his point is well-taken as a warning that the singlestate fallacy leads us to selectively restrict our 'mental instrument' to only one way of working. Remember the analogy in Chapter 8: Just as there are many different programs we can install in a computer, there are many different information processing programs — mindbody states — we can install in our minds

Mindbody State as Variable

In previous chapters we recognized improvements a multistate approach brings to our thinking: (1) if we survey all mindbody states, we can build a more complete map of our mind; (2) as psychomagnifiers, psychedelics allow us to experience parts of our minds in more detail than we otherwise could; (3) psychomagnifiers and other psychotechnologies point out the parameters we should pay attention to as we describe our cognitive and non-cognitive mental processes, and they widen our knowledge of the range these parameters can exhibit; (4) in our accumulations of knowledge (databases) in many disciplines, we too often fail to include information about other mindbody states (This gives us a standard for evaluating generalizations and theories.); (5) other mindbody programs can be useful, as in creative problem solving or healing (See Part 2 of this book.); (6) other kinds of intelligence exist in other states; (7) the ability to choose states, enter them, and access their resident abilities is a kind of background, executive, or metaintelligence; finally, (8) by extending our repertoire of mental skills, multistate abilities add to our mental flexibility, making individual people and groups more adaptable and competitive — possibly increasing survivability. These all have to do with finding knowledge and using it.

As a research instrument with many possible settings (information processing routines), we can select which programs to use, and the mind itself now becomes a variable. Not only can we do research *about* different mindbody states, but researchers may actually *use* several states. Will the most skillful future researchers use this instrument in widely diverse ways? Will using several mindbody states allow researchers to triangulate their investigations from several multistate perspectives?

The development of methods and techniques for doing multistate research remain one of the most difficult and intriguing areas for bright minds to play with.

Maybe I'm getting grandiose over this, but I believe that exploring and developing mindbody states can enrich most academic, scientific, and artistic fields. In my judgment it is the major intellectual opportunity of our times. Why?

Research Land Rush

Since there are hundreds of psychotechnologies which create wide-ranging mindbody states, each of these questions represents whole fields of potential research. For example, even if we were to limit ourselves only to the

---

THE CENTRAL MULTISTATE QUESTION

How does/do _____ vary from mindbody state to mindbody state?

To sample the opportunities that the Central Multi-state Question and its paradigm offer, try inserting the topics below into the question. To invent additional hypotheses, questions, and intellectual agendas, insert your favorite topics into the question.

cognition	*consciousness*	*movement*
meaning	*learning*	*memory*
language	*aesthetics*	*theology*
development	*emotions*	*perception*
performance	*sensations*	*observation*
values	*identity*	*reason*
motivation	*health*	*social interaction*
intelligence	*self-concept*	*etc.*

---

many forms of martial arts, or limited our questions to psychoactive drugs, or considered the numerous types of meditation, we'd frame thousands of research topics and invent almost endless opportunities for scientific and scholarly research.

Beyond looking at the things we might study and the questions we might ask, another set of opportunities arises. In experimental terminology, mindbody psycho-technologies and the states they produce can be both independent and dependent variables. When we compare thinking in our usual state with thinking during various psychedelic states, we change our state to see what the differences are. In this case mindbody state is an independent variable (we are intentionally changing it), and thinking is the dependent variable (its changes depend on which psy-

chedelic or other mindbody psychotechnology we use).
That is, we change mindbody state to see how that change
affects any of the topics (and others) listed in the Central
Multistate Question.

Given the enormous variety of mindbody psychotechnologies and the almost endless number of topics, the
multistate approach offers a practically endless frontier
for mind exploration. Not only that, but most of the topics
in the box are complex collections of many more specific
topics. Cognition, for example, isn't just one topic, but
looks at how all our mental processes occur. Similarly how
people change as they age (developmental questions) and
learning are complex fields of interlocking observations
and theories. Part 4 of this book on education illustrates
how the topics in that one discipline expand to include a
multistate perspective. Similar matrixes might be constructed for other disciplines too. People who like to
invent new agendas and frame new questions can have a
field day.

In addition to looking at how mindbody states affect
whatever interests us, we can study the states themselves,
the psychotechnologies that create them, and other influences on them. Here the states are dependent variables.
What states do LSD, mescaline, caffeine, nicotine, or
other drug psychotechnologies produce? How do states
produced by different forms of meditation differ from each
other, and how do they resemble each other? What states do
various forms of ritual dancing and chanting produce? How
should we go about describing them? Again, given the plen-
tiful supply of mindbody psychotechnologies and with new
ones being steadily invented and imported from other cultures, there is enough to keep decades of mind explorers
busy and generations of university researchers busy.

As I mentioned in the previous chapter, Benny Shanon's
excellent book *The Antipodes of the Mind* blazes a multistate
trail for future researchers to follow. As a cognitive psy-

chologist, Shanon describes the cognitive aspects that the Amazonian sacrament ayahuasca produces and its effects on thinking processes. By bringing ayahuasca and cognitive studies together, *Antipodes* sets a standard for systematically exploring 'programs in our mind'. More important than Shanon's specific findings about ayahuasca, *Antipodes* illustrates how researchers in cognitive studies might examine other mindbody psychotechnologies and the states they produce — the questions to ask, the observations to make, how to incorporate information from other people, and so forth. I expect *Antipodes'* long-term importance will be because it illustrates how to combine an existing academic area (here cognitive studies) with mindbody states (here ayahuasca).

Consilience

Another advantage of psychedelic research is that it is naturally interdisciplinary. It cuts across everything from biochemistry of our brains to Greek mythology and biblical history. Seeing how various levels of reality and of knowledge influence each other and fit together is a major problem in how we understand our world. Psychedelics help address this problem of integrating different lines of inquiry into a multi-layered scaffolding of empirical evidence and ideas. For example, how do the chemical, biological, psychological, cognitive, and social levels influence each other? Psychedelics provide ready experimental ways to look at such questions. With psychedelics the question, 'How do biochemical changes affect beliefs?' is open to experiments. Conversely, researchers can experimentally examine, 'How do someone's beliefs and cognitive set influence the outcomes of biochemical experimental treatments?' By providing ready models for independent variables on one level and dependent variables on others, meditation, psychedelics and other mindbody techniques naturally lend themselves to a multi-level approach. The intellectual project of integrating various levels — *consilience* as Edward Wilson calls it — is a major project for the sciences and humanities. Psychedelic studies — and other mindbody research too — provide ready-made roads for the consilience project to advance.

Are we on the verge of a sort of intellectual and scientific Oklahoma Land Rush? The lands of multistate research stand open to be explored. When they ask: 'What are our minds' fullest and most beneficial potentials?' explorers from many disciplines have the opportunity to plant the flags of their specialties in the newly opening multistate lands. Young scholars have astonishing opportunities to stakeout multistate specialties in their disciplines, broaden their disciplines' databases, formulate new questions, develop mindbody research methods, and take the lead in exploring and developing these topics. In our intellectual landscape, chess is not the only game in town.

Psychead —
Psychedelic Higher Education Association
— A Project

Invigorated by psychedelics, one of my favorite ideas is an association of professionals to share research on psychedelics and to organize a professional specialty. A Psychedelic Higher Education Association would draw from most academic, scholarly, scientific, and artistic fields. I like the nickname 'Psychead.' It would contract the name and manage a nice pun on 'psychedelic head.' Psychead's members — known as 'psycheads' — would come from higher education, research institutes, libraries, museums, scholarly and professional societies, and similar institutions. Psychead's purpose would be to exchange information on psychedelics and promote their research through publications, meetings, and other scholarly channels.

At first this might seem unrealistic or an idea whose future has yet to come; however, when I give papers on psychedelics at professional meetings, afterwards there typically are one or two people who confide in me about their interests in this field. Similarly, from time to time new professors from various departments drop by my office and admire my 60s rock posters. In a sentence or two we are talking about our mutual interest in the academic possibilities that psychedelics offer. But due to the censorship or self-censorship, these young colleagues feel they can't discuss this aspect of their professional interests. Colleges and universities are supposed to encourage the exploration of ideas wherever they lead, but these young faculty members are afraid to discuss what for many of them are their most challenging and intellectually intriguing experiences. This is a terrible situation to exist in an institution one of whose main principles is supposed to be open-mindedness and freedom of academic inquiry. Another job for Psychead would be to end this perception of persecution and its chilling effects on academic freedom by establishing professional academic standing.

Summary

In chapter 8 through this one, we've skimmed through a multistate paradigm. A new paradigm should:

(1) include new phenomena

(2) posit new relationships among them

(3) introduce useful concepts

(4) accept and help explain anomalies

(5) stimulate new research questions and directions

(6) provide new variables, treatments, and methodologies

(7) strengthen professional preparation.

The multistate paradigm does these. It includes observations about other mindbody states and their phenomena and processes. It proposes that the abilities we now have will be stronger in some mindbody states and weaker in others. Other abilities may show qualitative changes. The multistate paradigm introduces concepts such as 'mind-body psychotechnologies' and 'residency'. Multistate theory posits that some odd phenomena and rare abilities may be anomalous only because we judge them from our limited singlestate perspective. We may be able to invent new mindbody states, and — more speculatively — as we explore these states, we may even discover new, undreamed of abilities. The Central Multistate Question proposes expanding research agendas with questions such as 'How does cognition vary from mindbody state to mindbody state?' It makes mindbody state both a dependent and independent variable and gives us methods to explore how human abilities vary from state to state. At the same time, the multistate paradigm criticizes current professional education because it neglects mindbody states as it selectively and systematically omits significant information and methods. It multiplies future research possibilities. It offers future graduate programs the tasks of collecting knowledge about mindbody states from cultures worldwide, making new generalizations from these wider databases, and examining these findings to see how they might benefit us.

In Chapter 8 we started out this part of *Psychedelic Horizons* by looking at three basic questions of mind studies and education:

- What is the nature of the human mind?
- What is its fullest education?
- How do we achieve this?

Chapters 8–12 focused on the first question and tasted some appetizers from the second question. The next 2 chapters develop the second and third questions further, but Chapters 13 and 14 don't so much answer them as they point to systematic strategies for addressing them. Whatever our answers, they must acknowledge that we can produce and use many mindbody states. For the future, mapping the whole terrain of our minds' many states along the virtually endless mindbody horizon and developing these states' resident abilities invigorates both the disciplines that study our minds and the disciplines which use our minds. This doesn't omit much.

Remember again our imaginary friend who bought a new computer: chess is not the only game in town.

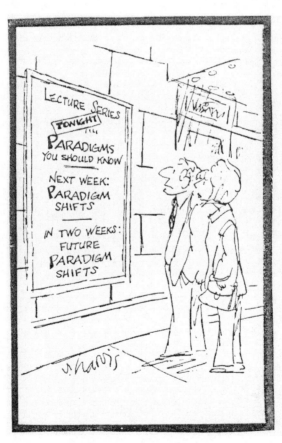

With thanks to Sidney Harris for
permission to print his cartoon.

PART FOUR

Enlarging Education

The first benefit was the simple recognition that there are realms of experience, modes of self, and states of consciousness far beyond the ken of our day-to-day experience or our traditional cultural and psychological models. These experiences were often said to produce expanded belief systems, making people less dogmatic and more open to as yet unexperienced or undreamt realms of being. One common report was that each experience tended to elicit a deeper realm and a more expanded sense of consciousness and self, so that the previously expanded belief system continued opening and widening.

For all five of the subjects mentioned here, and many of their students, psychedelic experience produced a new interest in depth psychology, religion, spirituality, and consciousness, as well as related disciplines and practices such as meditation. All the subjects believed that their psychedelic experiences enhanced their ability to understand these consciousness disciplines. In particular, the esoteric core of the great religions and spiritual traditions could be seen as roadmaps to higher states of consciousness, and some of the most profound material in these traditions became especially clear and meaningful during psychedelic sessions. ...

Most of the subjects felt that the psychedelic experience could sometimes supply a guiding vision which provided direction and meaning for one's life thereafter. They mentioned intense emotions such as love, compassion, or empathy, and the recognition that the mind can be and should be trained. Three subjects mentioned another residual benefit. Someone who has had a deep positive insight may be able to recall that insight subsequently and use it to guide himself or herself through a situation where it lends an additional useful perspective, even though it is no longer directly available.

Roger Walsh
Psychedelics and Self-Actualization (pp. 117–18)

Chapter 13

It Means Something Different to be Well Educated

To me, this short chapter is as important as the longer chapters but with more importance per word because it reframes 'well educated' from a multistate perspective.

How does/do _____ vary from mindbody state to mindbody state? The Central Multistate Question from the previous chapter changes the way we look at the fullest development of our minds, including current schooling, university, professional development — all learning throughout our lives. *What happens when we insert educational topics into this question?* In this chapter we'll see these two italicized questions as the grandparents of 8 families of questions, each with hundreds of offspring questions. The possibilities seem endless.

When we realize that there are hundreds of mindbody psychotechnologies, if not thousands, it's clear these two general questions unpack into thousands of specific questions — certainly too much to answer in one chapter of one book, in fact, too many to answer in many books. So rather than trying to answer these endless questions in this chapter, I want to show you a useful matrix I use to think about them and to organize them.

I developed the 'All the Questions Get Reasked' matrix (below) by imagining what might happen if I presented a multistate mindview to my colleagues in the College of Education at Northern Illinois University. What questions would they come up with?

Columns – Standard Research Questions

I thought about the instructional and research questions they typically would ask about how their specialties might intersect with each mindbody psychotechnology. Typically they would ask such questions as: 'What are the implications of meditative states for curricula?' or 'How would the martial arts influence various special education students?' and so forth. I think they would start by seeing psychotechnologies as instructional techniques (ways of teaching) to teach current knowledge and skills, only later as valuable cognitive skills to learn (content of teaching). The questions grouped themselves into 8 major areas of interest, and these became the columns of the matrix. So in reality, each column represents a large group of related questions and subquestions by the dozens.

Rows – Mindbody Psychotechnologies

My colleagues would want to know how each mindbody psychotechnology could intersect with each column and its questions and implied subquestions, so the psycho-technologies became the rows of the matrix. Actually, a full matrix would be much larger than the one below. Just as each column is a group of related questions and topics, each row actually represents a family of mindbody psychotechnologies; there are many kinds of mediation, hundreds of psychoactive drugs, and just as each column would divide into many specific questions, each row would too. A full list of all the psychotechnologies and their subtypes would be hundreds of rows long, so a

All the questions get re-asked — STANDARD RESEARCH QUESTIONS

Mindbody Psychotechnology	Literature research — What can be learned/known?	Taxonomy for each — What goals and objectives?	Developmental questions — How do age/stage effect these?	Measurement / evaluation questions — How to assess, evaluate, measure?	Methods and materials development — What methods, teach these?	Curricular questions — What place in the curriculum?	Sociological questions — How do ethnic / other groups vary?	Special education questions — Implications for gifted/disabled etc.?
Psychoactive drugs								
Meditation(s)								
Martial arts / yoga								
Hypnosis								
Dreams								
Relaxation / imagery								
Biofeedback								
Contemplative prayer								
Sensory isolation								
Sensory overload								
Breathing exercises								
Etc.								

matrix that included boxes for all questions and all psychotechnologies would be huge.

This matrix doesn't even look at different sequences and recipes of psychotechnologies. That would multiply the number of rows and boxes many-fold. And to make matters still more complex, many of the standard research questions from the Reasking Matrix and the questions from the Central Multistate Question in Chapter 12 may have different answers for different aged students.

The leading edge work of a doctoral student in education at the University of British Columbia in Vancouver, Canada, illustrates how the matrix provides a home for education's expansion and how it suggests new leads to follow. In 'Entheogens and Existential Intelligence: The Use of Plant Teachers as Cognitive Tools', Kenneth Tupper shows how entheogens — psychoactive plants and chemicals used in a religious context — support Howard Gardner's putative existential intelligence. One reason this intelligence is so hard to tie down may be because it is often associated with other mindbody states, and Tupper's work supports the idea that other kinds of intelligence may exist in other states. In 'Entheogens & Education: Exploring the Potential of Psychoactives as Educational Tools', Tupper proposes 'possible applications of entheogens … as potential educational tools to stimulate foundational types of understanding'. He is, in effect, suggesting that some day these psychotechnologies may become ways to enrich some standard educational practices.

Learning — A Comparison of Singlestate and Multistate Approaches

This table summarizes some of the adjustments that occur to education and mind development when we switch from a singlestate perspective to a multistate perspective. Again, MBS = mindbody state.

A Comparison of Singlestate and Multistate Paradigms

— Learning —

ASSUMPTIONS OF SINGLESTATE PSYCHOLOGIES	ASSUMPTIONS OF MULTISTATE PSYCHOLOGIES
Abilities/Capacities	
All valuable and learnable abilities reside in our ordinary MBS.	As one changes MBS, some abilities weaken or disappear. Others strengthen or appear anew.
Classical/Operant Learning	
It is impossible to control the autonomic nervous system voluntarily except by physical or chemical intervention. Classical conditioning is clearly different from operant conditioning.	It's possible to control the autonomic nervous system voluntarily by yoga, meditation, imagery, biofeedback, psychoactive drugs, and other mindbody psychotechnologies.
Memory	
Memory is most reliably developed, accessed, and studied in our usual MBS.	Psychedelics, meditation, dreams, hypnosis, and other mindbody psychotechnologies provide access to memories not readily available in our usual MBS.
Teaching/Learning	
The best ways of teaching and learning are in our usual MBS.	Many people learn best in MBSs such as relaxed imagery, etc.
Performance	
Peak performance is learned by repetitive practice of component skills.	Peak performance is correlated with MBS alteration.

Continued on next page

Continued from previous page

ASSUMPTIONS OF SINGLESTATE PSYCHOLOGIES	ASSUMPTIONS OF MULTISTATE PSYCHOLOGIES
Special Education	
Special education students are best understood as physically or behaviorally impaired and best improved by chemical intervention.	Some special education populations may be in different MBSs, so multistate teaching techniques may be the most appropriate instruction.
Moral Development	
The path of moral development leads from narrow self-interest to universal abstract principles. People learn this path from life experiences.	During self-transcendent MBSs, one can immediately apprehend non-ego centered moral principles and universal values, which guide moral action, social concerns, and global or cosmic standards.

Related Questions

Which mindbody psychotechnologies are not appropriate for schools, and which ones may have school uses? Which institutions might best develop non-school ones? Many of these possibilities would probably be handed better outside of formal schooling as we now know it, such as families, organizations for both youth and adults, churches, museums, libraries, Internet resources ... wherever people learn and develop. In 'Chemical Input, Religious Output,' I've looked at some of the potentials for religious organizations to increase spiritual intelligence.

'How do we achieve our minds' best and fullest potentials?' Whatever the answer is, it includes being able to use our abilities in many mindbody states. To reach this goal, we may have to use current organizations and institutions in new ways and found new ones. It seems obvious to me that no one person can produce and use all mindbody states. Just as we now have a variety of occupations, in the future we may have a variety of specialists who use various mindbody states.

How does our view of learning change when we use a multistate perspective? How might education advance when we employ the Central Multistate Question to think about learning? How does education vary from mindbody state to mindbody state? There are enough questions here to keep generations of researchers busy exploring the frontiers of mindbody learning.

Thank You, Psychedelics

As an educational psychologist, I am grateful to psychedelics for teaching me that our minds function in many mindbody states and that cognition, emotions, and even physical processes can vary so much. While I might have realized this by paying attention to sleep, dreaming, wakefulness, drunkenness, sleeplessness, caffinity, or many other states, it was psychedelics' jolt that awakened me. From psychedelic beginnings, I am exploring a variety of mindbody scholarship to investigate what our minds are capable of. The horizon still beckons. Psychedelics have prodded me to ask the questions in this chapter and in this book, to try to organize the challenges they present into some sort of order. As Roger Walsh phrased it in this chapter's epigraph, psychedelics have 'provided direction and meaning' to my life. They aren't the only source of meaning, of course, but they are a major influence. This book, as a fruit of these experiences, shows they have 'produced a new interest in depth psychology, psychology, religion, spirituality, and consciousness' and helped me wonder about things I otherwise would not have wondered about.

Following the psychedelic trail lead me to topics I doubt I would have otherwise investigated: the archeology and theology of ancient Greece, the origins of religion, the theology of mystical experiences, women's drug experiences, the politics of drug policy, the economics of prohibition, and related fields.

I am not saying that other people might not have followed the mindbody quest from other starting points or along other paths. Clearly they have. It isn't to say they wouldn't have asked the same questions. But in my life psychedelics challenged me to explore our minds, and I am thankful that they invited me when they did.

Basically, these questions in the Reasking Matrix blow the roof off educational research, practices, goals, and methods as we now know them. They direct our attention to new things we can know, the number of cognitive processes we can use, and add to the methods we have for learning to use our minds. In summary, they reformulate what it means to be a well educated person.

A well-educated person can select appropriate mindbody states, enter them, and use their resident abilities. The idea is simple enough; its achievement isn't.

The essential question then arises: What is the potential reward in exploring this unexpected experience, or is it something to be avoided? Exploration involves risk, but it also increases the acquisition of knowledge, and the brain's dopamine superhighway system is essential to both. This is confirmed by extensive research in primates, which has shown that new learning takes place when unexpected environmental changes occur [psychedelics? —TR] and the firing rate of the dopamine neurons increases. Thus, the dopamine superhighways (frequently called the dopamine 'reward' system, for obvious reasons) are what sustain our curiosity and bring novel events to the attention of the executive centers of the limbic brain and of the cerebral cortex for rapid assessment and action.

Peter C. Whybrow
American Mania: When More Is Not Enough (p. 64)

Chapter 14

Enlarging Learning

The increasing number of psychotechnologies is extending our view of what we can learn, what our minds are, and what it means to be a person. Carrying on the states/programs analogy from earlier chapters, like new programs for computers, mindbody programs make it possible to learn to do additional things with our minds, brains, and bodies. Examples abound. Through biofeedback people learn to control their autonomic nervous systems to an extent thought impossible a few decades ago. As a result, the psychomotor domain (learning that has to do with movement and bodily control) has expanded many times.

Meditation increases both the content learned and classroom behavior of students. Imagery seems to be especially powerful in other mindbody states and is used successfully in sports, as a technique for teaching subject matter content, and as a way to strengthen the placebo ability. Hypnosis raises questions about how one learns to be a good hypnotic subject and about the kind of memory that is tapped during these and other mindbody process.

As we saw in the previous chapter, ideas such as 'mindbody state,' 'mindbody psychotechnology,' and 'residency' expand the meaning of what it means to be a well educated person (now with multistate capacities):

A well educated person can select from a large number of mindbody states, enter them, and use their resident abilities. In this chapter, we will speculate about some future directions multistate education may take us: doing 'impossible' things, improving grad students' education, envisioning multistate mental health and enlarging counseling, psychedelic frontiers of Otherness, inventing new mindbody states and designing new cognitive processes, and, finally, a center for housing and promoting these advances.

Possibling the Impossible

When we think about a thinking process or bodily ability as being possible or impossible now, we need to remind ourselves to add 'according to what we now know about our ordinary mindbody state.' Some rare and unusual abilities may become more commonplace when we gain access the states where they presumably reside. When we learn to use our minds in new ways, the residency principle leads us to expect that we'll discover new abilities, changing what we think of as 'possible' and 'impossible.' And what we now know is constantly changing. With luck and courage, exploring our multistate capacities will release new possibilities.

Grad Students Dancing with Anomalies

Because anomalies are observations that contradict existing scientific theories, they are often ignored or even met with hostility. Sometimes they are simply oddities or errors, and the scientific community is correct in ignoring them. Sometimes scientists dismiss them as lying beyond the bounds of their fields of inquiry. Until recently anomalies having to do with other mindbody states were dismissed this way, but thanks to Thomas Kuhn's book *The Structure of Scientific Revolutions*, more scientists are coming to recognize anomalies' benefits to scientific thinking. They can spark scientific advances. They mark current theories' limitations. They alert researchers to possible errors; and they may turn into leads to future research directions. Recognizing anomalies and trying to make sense out of them is a good intellectual task for advanced students and may lead some of them to solve current problems or start new lines of research.

Where are the anomalies that can challenge our graduate students today? The multistate woods are full of anomaly trees. Practically any good book about research on hypnosis, meditation, psychedelics, or other altered states will provide enough anomalies to keep a whole class struggling intellectually and feasting conceptually. If these don't oil some rusty minds, the anomalies that research on parapsychology has documented will.

Although they prefer to present their research in terms of 'engineering anomalies' rather than 'parapsychology,' the anomalies captured by the Princeton Engineering Anomalies Research (PEAR) program would qualify as 'parapsychological' to most people. Among other paradigm-breaking anomalies, they have documented the ability of consciousness to affect the rate of decay of radioactive materials (psychokinesis) and the ability to send information over long distances (telepathy). Graduate students with a mind for mind exploration will enjoy exploring the PEAR website and reading its publications.

In their own words, PEAR studies 'concepts that generally seem to characterize conditions or situations in which we may expect an anomalous effect.' To me, most of the conditions they found resemble the ones that characterize different mindbody states, especially those we discussed in Chapter 7 that occur with spontaneous remission and the POTT MUSIC characteristics of mystical experiences:

Engineering and Consciousness

The Princeton Engineering Anomalies Research (PEAR) program was established at Princeton University in 1979 by Robert G. Jahn, then Dean of the School of Engineering and Applied Science, to pursue rigorous scientific study of the interaction of human consciousness with sensitive physical devices, systems, and processes common to contemporary engineering practice. Since that time, an interdisciplinary staff of engineers, physicists, psychologists, and humanists has been conducting a comprehensive agenda of experiments and developing complementary theoretical models to enable better understanding of the role of consciousness in the establishment of physical reality.

http://www.princeton.edu/~pear/

---

(1) Group resonance, particularly in emotionally meaningful contexts

(2) High ratios of subjective to objective, or emotional to intellectual contents

(3) Relatively profound personal involvement, especially if shared by a group

(4) Deeply engrossing, fully interactive communication

(5) Situations or sites that are spiritually engaging

(6) Circumstances that evoke a sense of fun and humor

(7) Activities that are inherently creative, and bring freshness or novelty for participants.

Emotionally meaningful, subjective and emotional, profound personal involvement, deeply engrossing, spiritually engaging, positive affect, creative, fresh, and novel — I don't know about you, but to me these sound like a pretty good description of standard psychedelic experiences. It looks like PEAR is on its way to discovering 'set and setting,' which are two of the three major variables determining the effects of psychedelics; the third is the drug itself.

There is disagreement over what extent parapsychological abilities reside in altered mindbody states. PEAR says these abilities reside primarily in our ordinary mindbody state, while other researchers such as Eysenck and Sargent say they are more characteristic of altered states. Here is a task for future multistate researchers. How do anomalous experiences and unusual abilities vary from mindbody state to mindbody state? Will teaching people to produce these states help them learn these abilities? There are enough new questions and reasked traditional questions here to keep a generation or more of educational researchers busy.

Revisioning Counseling and Mental Health

The table on page 178 shows how a multistate view reinterprets counseling and mental health.

The Psychedelic Frontiers of Otherness: External Otherness

A common trait in contemporary thought is a desire to experience and understand the 'Other.' Simply put, 'other' means people different from us and from cultures other than our own, but is this knowledge-seeking limited to just knowing about other people? I think this trait applies to novelty seeking of most kinds of curiosity, and, as the epigraph of this chapter implies, the dopamine systems in our brains reward new experience, increasing our knowl-

A Comparison of Singlestate and Multistate Paradigms

— Counseling and Mental Health —

ASSUMPTIONS OF SINGLESTATE PSYCHOLOGIES	ASSUMPTIONS OF MULTISTATE PSYCHOLOGIES
Anomalous Experiences	
Parapsychological, psychic, and related experiences are not real and are signs of error, perhaps mental illness.	Some anomalous experiences are associated with different MBSs and may be rare because we do not provide reliable access to the MBSs where they reside.
Abnormal Psychology	
Except for sleep and dreams, only our usual awake state is normal.	Achieving, exploring and developing MBSs is a healthy, normal human trait.
Personality Development	
Personality is learned through interaction with the environment from infancy on.	Personality also has roots in prenatal and perinatal development, possibly in sources beyond our usual MBSs.
Mystical, Oceanic, or Cosmic Experiences	
These are unimportant, irrelevant, and/or evidence of mental illness.	When properly integrated into the personality, they can be the most important therapeutic events in a person's life.
Psychotherapy and Counseling	
The goal of counseling is to help the client fit into existing society and overcome his/her personal problems.	An additional goal is to help develop his/her MBSs, transpersonal nature and spirituality.

Continued on next page

Continued from previous page

ASSUMPTIONS OF SINGLESTATE PSYCHOLOGIES	ASSUMPTIONS OF MULTISTATE PSYCHOLOGIES
Unconscious	
The unconscious is a source of mental illness and non-egoic thinking.	The ego and egoic thinking are functions of our ordinary MBS. Freud relegates all other MBSs and their mental functions to the unconscious; however, his methods of reaching the unconscious (dreams, hypnosis, relaxation, and imagery) are MBS psychotechnologies.
Trauma/Therapy	
One traumatic event can shape a life.	One intense therapeutic event can reshape it.
Alcoholism and Addiction	
These afflictions result from physiological and/or personality problems or are learned ways of coping with ego problems.	Addictions to substances, wealth, power etc. are ego attachments. In some cases these express unsuccessful attempts at ego transcendence.
Ego	
The ego has problems.	The ego is a problem.

edge. Are any experiences more packed with novelty than psychedelic experiences and other MBSs such as dreams? People who enjoy novelty, whether it's novelty of other people or other states, may have a genetically selected taste for newness and curiosity.

This gives us a natural curiosity about other people too. The more different they are, the more 'Otherness' they contain. Because these are qualities outside oneself, seeing people with different gender, language, sexual orientation, class, nationality, religion, and culture as Other is usually recognizing demographic and cultural differences as Other. These are sociological or anthropological approaches to Otherness, and psychedelics help us understand these external forms of Otherness when cultural explorers use different cultures' psychoactive plants or other mindbody psychotechnologies.

When they experience the mindbody states that host cultures use, these culture's ideas make more sense. Cultural explorer after cultural explorer report that the ideas and practices of ayahuasca-using Amazonian people made sense after they experienced the indigenous cultures' mindbody states. Thus, psychedelics and other mindbody psychotechnologies can help us understand the cultures that use them and ourselves.

A second benefit occurs when someone uses the mindbody states of the Other cultures to look back at our culture and ourselves.

> Oh wad some power the giftie gie us
> To see oursels as others see us.

Psychedelics sometimes grant Robert Burns's wish.

Psychedelic Frontiers of Otherness: Inner Otherness

As important as exploring other cultures' mindbody techniques are, psychedelics offer a much greater contribution to understanding Otherness than looking outward, more than exploring the world outside oneself. Psychedelics lead us to explore the Otherness frontier within. Inner, psychological explorations via psychedelics and other mindbody psychotechnologies are research methods for exploring inner Otherness.

First there is the hidden Otherness within oneself. This discovery occurs when psychedelic explorers uncover hidden thoughts, feelings, and experiences in their own minds that they had no idea were lurking there. These inner memories, fantasies, or creations are as foreign to one's sense of self as are their counterparts in the external world of other people and cultures. In fact, they are more surprising, and to some people frightening, because they are 'parts of me I didn't know about before.' They may include hidden fears, lost memories, created fantasies, or who knows what? To one's ordinary consciousness these are as foreign and sometimes as frightening as they are when discovered in other people. The inner discovery may be either frightening as when one discovers his own shadow, or they may be liberating and ecstatic, as when one discovers immense loving for others or for humanity or when one experiences 'the God within.' Sometimes having this experience occurs from the home base of one's self, or personal identity. Often this leads to transpersonal experiences. (See section below.)

During such experiences one's ordinary self (although altered with psychedelics) is doing the observing and reacting to the hidden, inner self or selves, so in this aspect the process is parallel to discovering Otherness in other people or their cultures. The self (or ego or identity) is still the center of consciousness, is still observing and reacting. In this sense, psychedelics (merely) extend one's observations and reactions inward: one's ego still does the observing. At other times, one's identity 'evaporates,' 'melts into a large whole,' or 'goes on vacation,' and transpersonal Otherness, as described in the following section, occurs

This second kind of inner Otherness occurs when one moves off the normal self as home base for observing other parts of one's mind and instead travels to these other parts and looks back. They ask: 'From these other parts of my mind, how does my self (identity) look?' During such experiences and when thinking about them afterwards, a psychedelically informed person can (but doesn't always) look back at his ordinary self and its normal thoughts, feelings, experiences, and world as Other. In this situation, one might reflect: 'I have an inner Other.' Or: 'I am my own Other.'

The Otherest Possible Experience?
Transpersonal Otherness

The very notion of Otherness supposes that there is a self which views the Other. That is, the self sees the Other and sees it as different, foreign, as not like oneself. But where there is no self, where is the Other?

Here is psychedelics' almost unique contribution to experiencing Otherness. They provide two entirely different ways of experiencing the Other. The first is discovering the transpersonal part of oneself, a radically new Other. The second comes from experiencing that the Other and self are the same; that is, one can directly experience unity between self and the Other.

During some psychedelic trips one may step outside himself or herself. I like to think of it as sending my usual identity, my usual self, 'on vacation.' Ecstasy — literally, standing outside oneself — is exactly the right word. This is the experience of going beyond the self, beyond the personal (trans-personal). In *The Doors of Perception*, Huxley refers to this as 'the blessed not-I.' In my mind I think of an imaginary 'Differentness Scale'. Some experiences are odd, a little bit different. Ones further along the scale are surprising, quite different, and those at the furthest end are completely unexpected, high in differentness. To me psychedelics can provide experiences that are anywhere along this imaginary scale. For me, my first mystical experiences were at the far extreme on this Differentness Scale.

Perhaps the thing I am most grateful for about my psychedelic experiences is discovering — experiencing — that religion *is* about something, and that something is unitive consciousness. It was edifying for me to discover that religion is based on real experiences, not just the millennia-long accumulation of ideas, historical accidents, and cultural accretions. In the chapter 'Chemical Input, Religious Output' I describe these experiences and the interdisciplinary intellectual adventures they've guided me to. A still untaught course I've designed *Entheogens – Sacramentals or Sacrilege?* resides on my faculty home page. These are further developments from *Psychoactive Sacramentals*, an anthology derived from a conference that was cosponsored by the Chicago Theological Seminary and the Council on Spiritual Practices. The conference-retreat included Huston Smith, Stan Grof, the Shulgins, Frances Vaughan, Roger Walsh, Charley Tart, among 30 others. Albert Hofmann and Brother David Steindle-Rast couldn't attend but contributed to the book. To me, the fact that so many important people attended the conference, took time away from their other duties, paid their own way, and expended the time and effort to write about their thoughts expresses the significance — sometimes supreme significance — people place on awakening to the spiritual aspect of their transpersonal Other.

Perhaps psychedelics' greatest contribution to understanding Otherness is providing a way most people can — with proper screening, training, and assistance — experience this far outpost of Otherness. This is definitely not to say that psychedelics are the only way to transpersonal Otherness, but they are probably the most efficient for most people. Other methods include contemplative prayer, various forms of meditation, biofeedback, breathing techniques, and spiritual practices from many cultures.

While LSD, mescaline, and their cousins have introduced me to inner Otherness, I have not tried DMT or ayahuasca, but from what Rick Strassman writes about DMT experiences in *DMT: The Spirit Molecule* and from what Benny Shanon says about ayahuasca in *The Antipodes of the Mind*, these chemicals sound even more Other than do my LSD experiences. According to their descriptions, these drugs put one's experience even higher in the Differentness Scale than LSD, mescaline, or peyote.

Both authors describe seeing beings that are not part of our consensual world and other bizarre phenomena that are beyond my psychedelic experiences. On the other hand, perhaps I am merely reporting the shallowness of my own experiences. In any case, psychedelics can provide lab-based, experimental Otherness, and from what I've experienced and read, these are Other to a greater degree than is meeting people from varied backgrounds and more different than soaking up other cultures. Psychedelics can (but do not always) provide a different kind of Otherness — 'another Other,' so to speak — not the Other one encounters while still standing on one's ego, but one in which I becomes Other. To return to our Central Multistate Question: How does Otherness vary from mindbody state to mindbody state?

Inventing Mindbody States

Exploring other states and developing their useful potentials is not the whole multistate story by a long shot. A distinct and generally unrecognized opportunity arises from a multistate paradigm. It is this: with a few exceptions, most mindbody psychotechnologies are used alone, one at a time. By combining psychotechnologies into novel recipes or by ordering them in new sequences, will it be possible to construct mindbody states which have not existed before? Personally, I find this idea the most intriguing one that psychedelics and other mindbody psychotechnologies bring to mind development. Can we go beyond discovering, describing, and domesticating mindbody states as they now exist to designing new states?

New psychotechnologies are increasing the number of ingredients available for designing new mind programs. For example, a decade ago, ayahuasca and ibogaine were almost unknown drug-based psychotechnologies. Now there are books and conferences devoted to them. *TIKAL* and *PIKAL*, two books by Alexander 'Sasha' and Ann

Shulgin list hundreds of psychoactive drugs that have yet to be explored for their educational and psychological potentials.

Anthropology is a steady source of both drug and non-drug psychotechnologies and promises to import more mind-development methods that are new to our culture. In *Religion, Altered States of Consciousness, and Social Change,* Erika Bourguinon, reports that 'of 488 societies, in all parts of the world, for which we have analyzed the relevant ethnographic literature, 437, or 90% are reported to have one or more institutionalized, culturally patterned form so altered states of consciousness.' Another way in which anthropology is a leader in mindbody studies is the Society for the Anthropology of Consciousness. As we move toward cultural diversity, we need to recognize that part of this diversity includes knowing which mindbody states various cultures use, their psychotechnologies for achieving them, how they think about these states, how they integrate them into their cultures, and what abilities may reside in them. The 'Dancing with Anomalies' section of this chapter picks up on this theme as a way to enrich graduate education.

The multistate paradigm provides a way to think of a new series of questions. What will happen if we invent recipes that combine, say, hypnosis, ayahuasca, and contemplative meditation? Will these recipes construct previously unknown states? What cognitive programs will appear in them? Which current abilities become stronger or weaker in them? Will new, different kinds of, say, intelligence appear? Will these researchers discover (or construct) new, presently unknown abilities? A multistate perspective encourages psychological and educational researchers to invent new cognitive processes. This is a new kind of scientific endeavor.

Clearly this is an area for extreme caution and ought to be investigated small-step by small-step by well trained and thoroughly competent professionals.

Designer Cognitive Processes

Where might designer cognitive processes take us? Beyond describing, educating, and using the mind merely as we now find it (a huge task on its own), the multistate paradigm gives us possibilities of designing minds as we would like them to be. To go back to the chess-player analogy from previous chapters, just as people are writing programs for computers which allow them to do things in addition to playing chess, will future mind designers invent new mindbody states that will allow us to do new things with our minds? I really don't know how to answer this question, but I know it's worth asking. Only the future will tell us where this mindbody form of technical innovation will take us. No, that's not quite right. Our decisions today will determine part of that future.

Every time humanity discovers a new power, the discovery raises ethical issues about how that power should and shouldn't be used. Just as advances in biotechnology and medicine raise a flock of ethical issues about what we should and shouldn't do with these new-found powers, parallel problems are beginning to arise from multistate mindbody powers. What states should and shouldn't be constructed? Why? Who gets to use them and for what purposes? Who gets to decide these issues? Each individual? Companies that patent new mindbody recipes? Governments? These may sound like questions for the far future, but current drug policy is raising them now in its arena. And as with electronic, bio-, and medical technologies, the ethical and political problems will multiply.

Center for Multistate Studies — A Project

In Chapter 8, 'Bigger, Stronger, Brighter,' I raised the possibilities of asking how our abilities vary from one mindbody state to others. In the last chapter we reasked the basic educational questions. Then we considered what I think of as 'The Mother of All Otherness' and 'mind design.' How might we systematically develop these leads, and how might other cultures contribute to this project? Finally, how might the speculations in this chapter be accomplished?

To start with, I think we need a systematic program to explore how current abilities vary across mindbody states, to reask educational questions from a multistate perspective, to explore leads from other cultures and our own, and develop the possibilities of designing new mindbody states and using them. The program needs to be housed somewhere — an Institute, Center, or Program for Multistate Studies. Such an institute would call on the various disciplines whose interests intersect with mindbody studies, from philosophy and religion to neuropharmacology and anthropology.

Two of the most profound ways cultures and subcultures differ are in the mindbody states and psychotechnologies they encourage and discourage. By teaching graduate students other cultures' preferred states and psychotechnologies, they would be better equipped to understand these cultures and may discover ways to enrich our own. A Multistate Center or Program would become truly international and multicultural in scope. Full multicultural studies would include other cultures' mindbody states and their ways of producing and using them.

As important as understanding other cultures is, there are far greater gains to come from a Center for Multistate Studies. I don't propose learning about other cultures' psychotechnologies merely to catalog them as cultural

> In recent years the West has begun to appreci-
> ate the fact that tribal societies can teach us
> much about the natural world from which we
> are so often alienated. It seems we may also
> have much to learn about the supernatural
> world, from which we are likewise alienated.
> Bearing in mind that humans have an innate
> need to experience altered states of con-
> sciousness, to ignore or repress our own
> natures in this way is to neglect our own
> capacities. What anthropology can do, by
> describing other cultures in which scientific
> and poetic approaches to truth are part of a
> holistic vision, is to remind us of the lack of har-
> mony in the elements of our own second
> nature. It can indicate ways in which we may
> reach a better understanding of the impor-
> tance of altered states of consciousness in
> both our collective and our personal lives.
>
> Richard Rudgley
> *Essential Substances in Society* (p. 175)

curiosities, not an updated version of nineteenth century
Orientalism. From a multistate perspective, knowledge of
other cultures' mindbody states and their psychotechnologies is primarily important because it will help us:

- draw a complete map of the human mind, including
  its full range of mindbody states
- discover unknown cognitive processes
- explore mindbody states as possible locations of
  unusual and rare skills
- develop the states and abilities which show promise
- learn how to use these mindbody psychotechnologies
  skillfully as research instruments, and
- add to the list of ingredients available for composing
  new mindbody states.

Graduate students in a Multistate Studies Center might do field work in Mexico to study peyote with the Huichols, travel to Thailand to practice Vipassana meditation, study Zen meditation in Japan, yoga in India, tai chi in China, ayahuasca in the Amazon, and so forth.

People tend to think of foreign students as studying American education to import American ideas and education back to their home countries. At a Center for Multistate Studies, intelligent recruiting would transform foreign students into teachers about the mindbody states and psychotechnologies of their homelands. Judiciously selected, they could be both visiting scholars and visiting students, and the Center would be a worldwide clearinghouse for mindbody skills. Will we someday have graduate teaching assistants or visiting professors from Thailand who teach mindfulness meditation classes to their fellow graduate students in, say, *Meditation 678: Advanced Methods of Mind Research*? Humanity would greatly benefit from a Multistate Center, and such an institute would open new frontiers throughout the world of learning. It would be a leader in developing our multistate minds' fullest education.

The same could be said of other fields of study too. Whether we are considering the philosophy of mind, religion, psychology, the sociology of mind, intellectual history, the neurosciences, or cognitive studies, such a center or institute would aid the humanities, sciences, arts, and professions by reframing their standard questions into a multistate framework. Academic disciplines would benefit from intellectual cross-fertilization and by filling in gaps in their current singlestate perspectives. They can complete themselves by including our minds' ability to achieve a range of mindbody states.

Summary

Our minds are more powerful than the singlestate view gives them credit for. When we realize we can learn to produce and use many mindbody states, then it means something different — something much more — to be a person, more to be a well-educated person. As we learn to use our minds in new ways, what will we discover about them? We can — if we strive — learn skills we now barely suspect exist. And we can — if we dare — invent new mental programs. 'What is our minds' fullest education?' 'How can we accomplish it?' These question-opportunities lead to unexplored frontiers, beckoning frontiers, educational frontiers.

Psychedelic horizons lead us to ask these questions and eventually go beyond psychedelic horizons to ask multistate questions along multistate horizons. But is this journey worth taking? Will we be better off from it? And where might it lead in the long run? Chapter 15 will speculate about these questions.

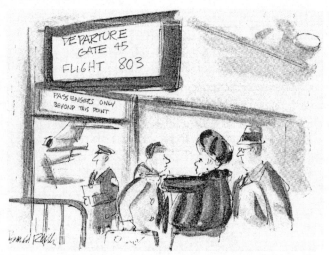

'Now be a good boy, study hard, and promise mother you won't go getting your consciousness expanded.'

With thanks to Donald Reilly for permission to reprint his cartoon.

Chapter 15

Is the Reprogrammable Brain Adaptigenic?

In this book we've seen how psychedelics provide us with ideas coming over the horizon, and we've seen that psychedelics are just one family in the larger tribe of multistate psychotechnologies that are changing our view of our minds, and consequently, our view of ourselves. What is true for psychedelics is even truer for the whole psychotechnology tribe. As a 'different book about psychedelics' in *Psychedelic Horizons*, we've only touched on psychedelics' better known uses, psychotherapy and religion, in order to emphasize some of their less obvious implications.

Religion and psychotherapy are certainly important and are significant parts of the psychedelic/multistate tapestry that our current culture is weaving. After years in hibernation, the psychotherapeutic uses of psychedelics is awakening and growing fast. The best up-to-the-minute source of information on this that I know and the one I consult is the research file at the website of the Multidisciplinary Association for Psychedelic Studies. New information appears there and elsewhere at the MAPS website several times a month. Another reason I'm not

writing about psychotherapy here — other than psychedelics' speculative possibility as a way to boost the
immune system — is that Michael Winkelman, a professor
of anthropology at Arizona State University, and I are
editing a pair of volumes *Hallucinogens and Healing*, which
is due in 2007. It will cover psychedelics' medical and
psychotherapeutic uses from addictions and alcoholism to
psychiatric and hospice psychotherapy. Researchers are
exploring these medical uses now in legally approved
pilot and clinical studies. Even though the religious uses
of psychedelics lags behind their therapeutic uses, I'm
including them in 'Today's and Tomorrow's Horizons'
because entheogens are making public appearances and
showing up in the press from time to time.

Today's and Tomorrow's Horizons

Using Disney's movie *Snow White* as an example, we've
considered psychedelics as a way to understand the arts.
The *Snow White* chapters sample Grofian psychocriticism,
which might be used not only throughout the arts, but also
in the social sciences and humanities. For example, in 'The
Perinatal Roots of Wars, Totalitarianism, and Revolutions,' Stan Grof has used his theory as a way to understand some psychological aspects of these historical
events. In 'Sartre's Rite of Passage' Riedlinger illustrates
how to use these psychedelic-based ideas to analyze
philosophical works. The leads for future critical and ana-
lytical studies are practically endless.

In the more speculative chapters on the immune systems, we noticed a common psychological shape between
psychedelic peak experiences, spontaneous remission,
and spiritual healings, and we wondered whether they
might all work via boosting the immune system. This possibility calls for psychological-biological-religious teams
of investigators. The words *wholeness*, *healing*, and *holy*
spring from the same root, and here is a chance to reunite

them. Just as we, Grof, and Riedlinger discovered similar (perinatal) psychological morphology in the current version of a popular folk tale, selected political/historical movements, and philosophy, we discovered another set of similarities among some instances of unusual healing and psychological events. Psychedelics seem to allow us to stand back and notice such similarities and make connections that otherwise would have escaped our notice.

That same ability to recognize parallels helped us see that many things that are true of psychedelics apply as well to the larger group of psychotechnologies, and just as it's important for psychology to include information about all mindbody states to be complete, the same standard applies to other fields of study. Psychedelics are a key to a much bigger intellectual house, and tomorrow's work for scholars and scientists includes following multistate leads. The Central Multistate Question blows the roof off many academic disciplines for they are artifacts of our little singlestate minds, and the multistate mind offers much more.

As if those of us in the mind-development vocations — educators — didn't have our hands full with trying to teach our students to use their minds skillfully in their ordinary, awake mindbody states, recognizing our minds' multistate capacities multiplies our task (and our opportunities) many fold. Whether we are talking about an Advanced Center for Multistate Studies or teaching kindergartners centering techniques, there are more than enough multistate leads for developing all aspects of intelligence.

Beyond our views over today's psychedelic horizons, lie other days and further vistas. As I mentioned in Chapter 1, as a thinking-intuitive type, I like to look forward and speculate about the global, long-term implications of things, so if you'll indulge me that proclivity a little more, let's look at some ideas that are approaching near-term then some that may be coming over the day-after-tomorrow's horizons.

Increasing Spiritual Intelligence

As I was rewriting and polishing this manuscript, Patrick McNamara, a professor at Boston University's School of Medicine, asked me to contribute a chapter to a 3-volume set of books he's editing on the brain and religion. Because the Central Multistate Question in Chapter 12 and the 'All the Questions Get Reasked' matrix in Chapter 13 have their parallels in religious studies, my writing grew beyond the limits of a chapter, but, fortunately, McNamara's publisher liked the ideas, and asked me to expand it into a book manuscript. I may be doing so as you read this. The gist of my chapter is that entheogens — both psychedelic and other psychoactive ones — advance religious studies beyond the limits of historical, anecdotal, descriptive, and correlational research to experimental studies. In other words, this picks up this book's theme and extends it to using psychedelics in religious settings. You can read a preview of *Increasing Spiritual Intelligence — Chemical Input, Religious Output* as well as up-to-date findings on neurotheology in McNamara's 3-volume set.

> **Interviewer:** *How do we reconcile this visionary experience with religion and with scientific truth?*
>
> **Albert Hofmann:** It is important to have experience directly. Aldous Huxley taught us not to simply believe the words, but to have the experience ourselves. This is why the different forms of religion are no longer adequate. They are simply, words, words, words, without the direct experience of what it is the words represent.
>
> *From Molecules to Mystery*

Democratizing Primary Religious Experience

The second gist of my chapter — if there is such a thing as a 'second gist' — is the question of whether we are now going through a transition in Western religion similar to the one that occurred around the year 1500. As I see it, for the ordinary person, the printing press and movable type opened up religious activity from primarily taking part in ceremonies to word-centered activities such as reading, writing, creeds, doctrines, beliefs, and other verbal activities. Printing democratized access to text, and religion became more oriented toward words than oriented toward ceremonies. Now we live in word-centered, thought-based religion, not rite-based. For example, to find out about someone's religion, we ask about cognitions, not practices. We ask: 'What do you believe?' not: 'What rites do you perform?' In a parallel move to the printed word 500 years ago, entheogens, it seems to me, democratize access to primary religious experiences, to mystical experiences. For example, for spiritual guidance, verbalists consult the word of God: mystics consult their experience of God. For the day after tomorrow's horizon, all the religious questions get reasked too.

Neuroplasticity

One of the unexpected findings in recent research on the brain is that parts of the brain that are repeatedly stimulated grow. First, the existing neurons grow stronger. Second, they grow additional branches out to other cells, both nearby and farther away (distance in cranial terms). Third, with additional use, the active parts of our brains grow new cells and may even invade adjacent areas of the brain and take over any unused space. This and similar growth processes are called variously 'cellular plasticity,' 'cerebral plasticity,' or 'neuroplasticity.'

When physical abilities, thoughts, and feelings strengthen, presumably the corresponding parts of our brains have strengthened too: as the part that controls, say, the left hand, grows, so does our ability to use our left hands. Presumably, our skills, cognitive processes, and emotions are the outward behavioral expressions of these inner biological structures. A corollary of 'Use it or lose it' becomes 'Use it and strengthen it.'

Under most circumstances, the active parts of our brains grow slowly, and our behavior, emotions, and thinking parallel this slow progress over time. Changes that occur over years, say, through playing a musical instrument or possibly through meditation, presumably fit the slow development path. But how do we account for changes in behavior and/or cognition such as those that follow sudden, overpowering experiences such as mystical experiences? Is there also a quick-development path? Rapid changes in our behavior, thinking, and feelings do occur. How are we to account for them? Presumably, there must be parallel changes in our brains too.

Mystical experiences (whether drug induced or occurring other ways) often cause major and permanent changes in people's thoughts, behavior, and beliefs. Are they a powerful fertilizer hastening rapid growth in various parts of our brains? If, over time, mystical circuits become more complex and larger through one powerful experience or many smaller ones, does it become easier to have mystical experiences more often or perhaps stronger ones? Here is a rich vein for entheogenic researchers to mine: how do peak experiences, mystical experiences, and their unitive-consciousness kin affect our brains? Why the sudden realignment?

The Day-after-Tomorrow's Horizons

Beyond the opportunities and problems coming over the horizon for our metaphorical todays and tomorrows, future days bring future horizons. Are we headed toward brain design? What ethical problems do we need to consider? Some of these are current; some lie in the future.

What institutions might best house psychedelics for which different uses, and how can we contribute to this process? Will we be insightful enough to use our new capacities wisely? Will the reprogrammable brain help us adapt to the world by enhancing our mental capacities? What may be coming over the horizons of our days-after-tomorrow? Here we'll speculate about some of these, and it might be helpful to consider some of them as science fiction and business fiction.

Designer Neurotransmitters and Designer Brains?

Personally, I'm not at all sure what to think of these possibilities, but they're ones we have to start thinking about. Looking at the trends of biological sciences, it's clear that we are steadily learning more about our brains' structures and functions. This includes how genes influence brain growth and development. We may soon be at the stage when we can turn on and off various genes (or other biological processes) that construct and maintain our brains.

So far most of the thought on this topic has to do with treating medical problems such as Alzheimer's or Parkinson's. The enhancement of brain/cognitive processes has recently received additional thought. Both the medical and cognitive orientations think about our brains only as they already exist, and they examine ways of improving our brains' normal functioning. And these are worthy goals.

However, as our knowledge of brain-building increases, our ability to influence and control them will increase too. Someday will we be able to, say, increase the volume of neurotransmitters a cell can produce or increase or decrease the number of receptor sites across the synaptic cleft? This seems likely to me. But let's go a step further into neurological science fiction. Will we develop the skills to design genes so that they produce new varieties of neurotransmitters and/or new kinds receptor sites to receive them? At some point in the future, will this go beyond merely improving what we now have and become a science of brain design, perhaps with wholly new transmitters and receptor sites? Cell design is on the way. If so, plants and chemicals that activate these sites will become newly psychoactive.

I have no idea where to go with this idea, but it's not too early to consider it.

> NEUROARCHITECT: Good morning, ma'am. How would you like your baby's brain designed?

Another psychoactive biotechnology frontier may exist in transplanting the genes that produce psychoactive compounds from one plant to another. Molds impress me as the most likely candidates. Using ergot, perhaps, or psilocybin mushrooms, is it feasible (or might it soon be) to transfer the genes that produce psychoactive compounds into currently nonpsychedelic hosts, say, blue cheese, other mushrooms, yogurt, or wine yeasts? What plants might hybridize with cannabis and adopt genes for making THC?

> UNIDENTIFIED STREET PERSON: Hey, man! I scored some dynamite blue cheese today. Want a hit?

Will the meaning of 'cheesehead' come to mean more than 'someone from Wisconsin'?

Multistate Bioethics

Just as current advances in medical knowledge and technique bring difficult ethical problems — abortion, stem cells, brain death, euthanasia, genetic selection, brain enhancement — future advances in mindbody biology and medicine present us with a store of problems. Before listing some of these, it's worth noting that today's controversial issues in bioethics include mindbody aspects which we often miss because we are weak both conceptually and cognitively (we have few appropriate concepts for multistate issues). We are weak in our ability to address the consciousness/mindbody aspects of these questions. To me, this is one reason these dilemmas are so intractable. Abortion, brain death, euthanasia, and brain enhancement all are partially mindbody or multistate issues; underlying these and other bioethical issues are the difficult questions: 'How do we define "consciousness" in other mindbody states? Do we define what it means to be a human solely by what that means only in our ordinary, awake state of consciousness? How do we adjust our ethical positions if part of human nature is the ability to produce a variety of mindbody states yet medical processes produce some states or terminate others?' I'm glad I don't have to answer these questions. I'll gladly leave them to the expertise of bioethicists.

Interviewer: *Do altered states implicitly convey something about ethics? Do they teach people to live more ethical lives?*

Michael Harner: Experiencing an altered state that occurs in the Middle World [our world of ordinary daily life] would not necessarily do that. However, outside the Middle World, the shamanic state of consciousness gets you in touch with the teachings of the compassionate spirits. These are concerned about reducing pain and suffering, and do indeed make it more difficult for you to be unethical. It's not that you can't be unethical, but you're going to have a harder time being unethical.

Tribal Wisdom: The Shamanic Path

What are the questions that multistate bioethicists need to consider? As with medical bioethics, they overlap.

• How might multistate theory contribute to current bioethical discussions?

- Do states other than our usual states of wakefulness, sleeping, and dreaming have value? What are their values, and what are their dangers? Which should we encourage? Which should we discourage?

- Some meditators and mystics claim the states they achieve are superior (perceptually clearer, conceptually subtler, morally elevated) to our usual state. If values vary from mindbody state to mindbody state, which state shall we select to make ethical judgments from? Why?

- What are we to make of the shift in values during states of unitive consciousness, both nonpsychedelic and psychedelic, away from personal, egocentric gains toward valuing social goods and cosmic standards?

- Do people who have achieved unitive states have a moral duty to influence others? Are they, in effect, morally better informed, more motivated toward higher goals?

- How should we evaluate knowledge about human nature and philosophy if the observations they are based on omit observations about other mindbody states?

- Because mindbody topics open broad opportunities within many academic disciplines, how do we decide where academic freedom collides with social mores, say, with current drug prohibition laws? Where does an academic's duty lie?

- To what extent does each person have a right to decide what goes on in his or her own brain and mind? Where does corporate responsibility lie?

- At what age are people competent to make these decisions about themselves?

- I'm not sure what to do with this one, but here it is anyway: If we gain access to a state where telepathy resides, is it an invasion of personal space to read someone else's thoughts? Given the advances in 'reading the brain' within medical technology, say in criminal cases, this issue is part of medical bioethics now. From a mindbody perspective, where does privacy begin and end?

- Behind most of our ethical considerations is the question of what happens to each person, but these judgments assume individual personhood, individuality, an egoic mind and existence. How do we rethink these topics if we recognize that individuality (the separateness of each person) is an artifact of one's mindbody state? How do transpersonal states reformulate these questions?

- To meet the standard of 'best evidence,' should bioethicists alter their mindbody states to be better informed of these issues? If they don't, how credible are their thoughts? If they do, how credible are their thoughts?

- Do people who haven't experienced various mindbody states even know what they are talking about? How can we have meaningful dialog among mutually uninformed people?

- If some mindbody states are conducive to healing, is it immoral to forbid them? (See EMXIS chapters in this book.)

- Are these issues legal, medical, religious, constitutional, human rights, political, economic, or what? It seems to me the answer is 'All of the above.'

- Who has the knowledge, moral authority, legal power, and individual right to make these decisions, to answer these questions? How do we handle conflicts when, say, knowledge and power disagree?

These are some menu items for a bioethicists' mindbody feast.

Community Psychedelic Centers, Inc.

In this book we've considered some opportunities that psychedelics and other mindbody psychotechnologies present for our institutions of healthcare, science, learning, and to a lesser extent religion. Once we start thinking with multistate ideas, these naturally fall into place. There is another institution that is less obvious, but seems to me to provide a faster, more powerful way of accelerating our speed in adapting a multistate view of ourselves and society. This is the free enterprise system, a business model. In an unpublished manuscript written as if it were a prospectus for an initial public offering of stock, I have designed an imaginary company whose service could be providing psychedelic sessions — screening, preparation, session guidance, and follow up and all that well run sessions require. Community Psychedelic Centers' business would not come primarily from manufacturing the drugs as many of them are off-patent or not patented in the first place, but from providing the sessions. (In the future, new psychedelics are likely to be synthesized, of course, and be patentable.). This company would be similar to companies which provide psychiatric or other services.

Because my plan is for a public stock company, in addition to being a business, the company would serve as a conduit for thousands, tens of thousands, or even hundreds of thousands of people around the world to combine their resources and coordinate their interests in psychedelics. Many people already know about psychedelics from their own experiences, others from the experiences of people they know, and still others from their reading about psychedelics without firsthand experience. They know about psychedelics' possible therapeutic effects, as aids in creative problem solving, and as a way of raising spiritual intelligence, so they might well see Community Psychedelic Centers as a worthwhile speculation.

However, more people are more interested in profits than in psychological growth. They want to know whether they could make money in Community Psychedelic Centers, Inc; these people outnumber people who are already informed about psychedelics. An initial public offering of stock would alert many people and encourage parts of the financial community to become informed about the research on psychedelics as part of their due diligence, thus spreading accurate knowledge about psychedelics and possibly recruiting powerful segments of society. Then, if investors, venture capitalists, mutual funds, banks, pension funds, endowments, and insurance companies bought, or were given, LSDD stock (my imaginary trading symbol), they would become advocates of responsible psychedelic research and encourage its responsible applications.

After they read the prospectus and exercise due diligence, some investors are likely to see they could benefit one way or another from well structured psychedelic sessions in a safe environment, benefit from the service their company provides. Sweet irony: greed would attract them to psychedelics in the first place, then their mystical experiences would free them from this egoic addiction.

At this point, I envision a company with two divisions, one for psychotherapy and the other for personal development such as problem solving, academic research, spiritual development, and creativity. Because much of the drug discovery process has already been accomplished, safety testing started or established, and small scale pilot studies in-process, Community Psychedelic Centers would start further along the process of corporate development than many startup medical technology and pharmaceutical companies. The money raised by an initial public offering would be used to fund further research on safety and efficacy to establish a strong database before applying for approval from various regulatory agencies worldwide.

While it's tempting to think the U.S. Food and Drug Administration would do everything it could to block such a company (at least until they see the data), there is no reason to suppose that the United States must be the home base of such a company. A parallel already exists with medical marijuana. G. W. Pharmaceutical's home is in England. I keep wondering about India with its strong mystical tradition and knowledge of soma or maybe even parts of Europe where its historical tradition of transcendent Christianity survives.

Is the Reprogrammable Brain Adaptigenic?

In Chapter 11 we spotted some survival advantages that mental adaptability and a wider range of behaviors confer, and in the epigraph to this book Grof claimed: 'It is my belief that a movement in the direction of a fuller awareness of our unconscious minds will vastly increase our chances of planetary survival.' Why did he say that? Does the information in this book confirm his optimistic claim? Do psychedelics (and by implication other mindbody psychotechnologies) support this hope? Yes, for several reasons:

First, psychedelics draw our attention to aspects of our world that we otherwise might miss, and a more complete view of reality certainly increases our chances of surviving and thriving.

Second, psychedelics give us a more complete view of our minds. Everything we perceive, feel, do, and think uses our minds, so the more we know about our collection of mind tools, the better we can use them.

Third, like additional programs in a computer, psychedelics provide additional information processing routines in our brains.

Fourth, by presenting us with psychedelic and psycholytic therapy, psychedelics help clear our minds of mental rubbish accumulated over our personal lives. Psychological rubbish warps our perceptions of reality, distorts our feelings, alters our reasoning, and makes us dysfunctional in other ways.

Fifth, by drawing our attention to the perinatal level of our mind, psychedelics help us recognize the short perinatal fuse (notably Grof's BPM II and BPM III) that is so easily ignited making us unconsciously willing to be violent and susceptible to war. This insight gives us perspective on ourselves, our times, and our political leaders, helping us become more resistant to bellicose feelings and war propaganda that our society and our leaders intentionally and unintentionally provide.

Sixth, related to this, we can recognize the perinatal roots of recreational violence, which so permeates human nature and our culture — movies, TV shows, news broadcasts, stories, violent sports. As we experience the perinatal parts of our minds and become aware of them, we can discharge their influence on us.

Seventh, experiencing and recognizing the transpersonal aspects of our minds reduces our egocentrism and greed. These keep us from helping others and expressing the care-giving that the social gospels of all the world's major religions instruct us to express in our lives. As Grof's quotation states: 'Deep reverence for life and ecological awareness are among the most frequent consequences of the psychospiritual transformation that accompanies responsible work with non-ordinary states of consciousness.' Or, as psychologist of religion, David Wulff expresses it:

> Among the predictable characteristics of mystical experience are a sense of the sacredness of all life and a desire to establish a new, more harmonious relationship with nature and with other human beings. There is a corresponding renunciation of the various forms of self-seeking, including the ethos of manipulation and control.

What might this mean to the future of humanity? Can psychedelics make us more moral? Used wisely, apparently so. If we fail to transcend our egos and misuse psychedelics and other psychotechnologies for personal gains, group power, or national aggrandizement, I am pessimistic. In hopes that we will extinguish the destructive and violent aspects of our minds (items 5 and 6) without giving up perseverance and achievement and in hopes that we'll practice more loving kindness toward others and our environment, I am excitedly optimistic about a psychedelically blessed human future. That future depends on what we do today.

Eighth, for the academic world psychedelics expand practically all the sciences and humanities into new directions. Not only do they direct our attention toward mindbody states as something to study, they also provide ideas for understanding ourselves and interpreting our cultures, e.g., the Snow White chapters in this book. They mentor us on how to ask new questions, frame new research agendas, and invent new specialties.

Ninth, psychedelics expand what it means to be a human. Now we become multistate.

Tenth, psychedelics expand what it means to be fully educated to include the skillful use of all useful, mindbody states and their resident abilities.

Eleventh, psychedelics provide a technique for problem solving and inventing.

Twelfth, psychedelics provide us with new cognitive processes and ways to invent still newer ones by sequencing mindbody psychotechnologies and combining them into new recipes.

Thirteenth, contributing to intergroup understanding, psychedelics increase our understanding of other cultures' ways of exploring their minds and using mindbody techniques.

Fourteenth, psychedelics provide novel psychotherapeutic treatments for a range of medical and psychotherapeutic problems. Of course, this is attracting attention
and is widely known, so I won't elaborate on this whole
flock of leads.

Fifteenth, psychedelics' uses for spiritual growth are
becoming more recognized, as the section 'Increasing Spiritual Intelligence' (above) points to.

From Foreword to Forward

A humanity composed of individuals who have a more
complete grasp of reality is likely to continue to thrive and
survive. A humanity with a wide range of cognitive skills
is better off than one with limited cognitive means. A
humanity which diminishes aggression, greed, and
mutual destruction, and one that promotes cooperation
will, as Roger Walsh writes in this book's Foreword, 'be
able to navigate our way through our current global crises.' A humanity that works toward the fullest development of its members will thrive. Setting a cautionary yet
hopeful tone for this book, Walsh continues:

> To achieve this, however, will require develop-
> ment of our mental capacities and inner world
> as much as our outer one. The challenge of
> realizing the possibilities of mind is no longer
> an academic question but an evolutionary
> imperative. Clearly we are in a race between
> consciousness and catastrophe, the outcome
> remains unsure, and we are all called to
> contribute.

We use our minds in everything we do, what we think,
the cognitive processes we think with, what we learn,
what we assume we can know, what we expect of ourselves and others. Our arts, technologies, sciences, lan-

guages, customs, relationships, laws, cities — all these are artifacts of our minds. When our view of our minds changes, our view of all these change too. So does the future. As the loudest of the mindbody psychotechnologies — the one whose voice we cannot ignore — psychedelics shout to us to change our view of our minds' capacities from singlestate to multistate — to recognize that we can do more with our minds than we have previously dreamed of. Thanks to the mindbody psychotechnologies — especially psychedelics — what it means to be a human is expanding.

*   *   *

I hope you've enjoyed my
little book of big ideas.

Good night.
Sweet dreams.

— Tom Roberts, INTP

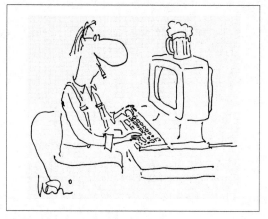

Chapter Notes

Full publication details of sources are in the Bibliography

Chapter 1: Psychedelic Horizons — Beyond Tripping

p. xvi   Epigraph: The quotation from Robert F. Kennedy can be found at http://www.brainyquote.com/quotes/quotes/r/q121273.html

p. 1   Charles Hayes (ed. 2000).

p. 2   Stanislav Grof (1975). *Realms of the Human Unconscious*. Grof refines and recapitulates his map of our minds in several of his subsequent books.

p. 4   Thomas B. Roberts (ed. 2001). *Psychoactive Sacramentals*.

         Isabel Briggs Myers and Katherine Cook Briggs. *Myers-Briggs Type Indicator*.

p. 5   Portentousness: Freedman (1968).

Chapter 2: Sometimes It's Lucky to be a Professor

p. 16   Epigraph : Joseph Campbell: (1949).

p. 20   Stanislav Grof: See the notes for the next chapter

         Joseph Campbell (1949).

p. 21   Joseph Campbell (1982).

p. 22   C. G. Jung (1973).

p. 24   Alan Watts (1963).

Chapter 3: Snow White — Grof's Landmarks in Disney's Land

p. 29   Epigraph: Stanislav Grof (1975). I expect *Realms of the Human Unconscious* to be recognized as a key book in Western civilization for 2 reasons.
         First, when a new scientific instrument is invented, it

often advances the sciences as new experiments using the invention provide us with information. *Realms* qualifies as one of the great books because in it Grof illustrates how to use psychedelics as a method of mapping previously obscure parts of our minds. As psychomagnifiers — ways of examining our minds in more details — psychedelics let us gain a more detailed picture of our minds. In this psychedelics are parallel to the microscope in biology and medicine and parallel to the telescope in astronomy, cosmology, and space travel. I elaborate on these ideas in chapters 8 and 11.

Second, we use our minds in everything we do, our thinking, emotions, actions, perceptions, and sensing. Furthermore, our expectations for what we can learn and can know depend on our view of our minds and their capabilities. Thus, when our ideas about what our minds are capable of change, this idea dominos into everything else we do. In *Realms* and his subsequent books, Grof presents an expanded view of our minds' potentials. What Grof found profoundly changes the way we see our minds. Naturally, this map expands our expectations for ourselves and for humanity; as such it represents a growth point in human history.

p. 39 Schultes (1976), pp. 25–26.

p. 41 In Eastern religions, mantra is the use of a sound as an aid in spiritual development, mudra the use of a movement or posture.

Tom Wolfe (1968).

Additional Bibliography to Chapter 3

I would like to thank Tom Lyttle, editor of *Psychedelic Monographs and Essays*, for contributing to this bibliography. An earlier form of this chapter first appeared in *PM&E* and later in Tom's book *Psychedelic Essays* (1994).

Peter Bishop (1981).

Jonathan Cott (1973).

Roberts Graves (1948). Graves speaks of the 'German folk-story Snow White' on p. 348.

Stanislav Grof (1980).

James Hillman (1974, 1977).

C. G. Jung (1966)

C. G. Jung (1973). The chapter The Phenomenology of the Spirit in Fairytales is especially relevant.

C. G. Jung (1976). Several excellent accounts of fairy tale symbology.

Jeremy Pascal (1981).

Thomas B. Roberts (1986). A Grofian analysis of the movie *Brainstorm*.

Barbara Stanford (1972).

Robert Warshow (1964).

Harry Wilner (1977).

Chapter 4: A Thinking Project

No notes on this chapter

Chapter 5: Binker's Stoned Idea

p. 53 Bicycle Day™ I have trademarked 'Bicycle Day'. It is available free to not-for-profit organizations and for non-commercial purposes.

p. 55 Albert Hofmann (1980).

p. 56 John Horgan (2003).

p. 57 Julie Holland (ed. 2001).

p. 59 Placebo ability: Roberts (1987). Is There a Placebo Ability? *Advances: Journal of the Institute for the Advancement of Health*. Vol. 4, No. 1, page 5 (letter to the editor):

'The discussion about the value of the placebo concept in the letter column of the Summer 1986 *Advances* misses an important point. Much of the problem associated with the concept stems from the phrase 'placebo effect.' This phrase is both illogical and a misnomer, and it serves to perpetuate ignorance about the so-called placebo effect.

A placebo treatment is selected because of its *lack of effect*. To attribute a change to a placebo is illogical. How can something that is chosen for its lack of effect be said to cause an effect?

I recommend that the phrase 'placebo ability' be substituted for 'placebo effect.' This would have the desirable result of encouraging research into this ability, just as we now investigate other human abilities such as cognition and creativity. It would stimulate a new set of research questions: Can one learn 'placebo-ing'? How can it be taught? What groups (of age or personality or ethnicity) are skilled or unskilled at this ability?

I do not intend to imply that current approaches to placebo be abandoned, only that additional directions of

investigation are possible and may result in a more complete understanding if one examines the placebo ability.'

Chapter 6: Do Entheogen-induced Mystical Experiences Boost the Immune System? Psychedelics, Peak Experiences, and Wellness

p. 65   J. Smyth et al. (1998).

For a good discussion of exceptional healing, see Krippner and Achterberg (2000). The book also includes a chapter on mystical experiences.

p. 66   *PubMed* is at http://www.ncbi.nlm.nih.gov/entrez . In my estimation, it must be one of the best uses of taxpayers' money in the government.

p. 67   A. A. Stone et al. (1996).

H. B Valdimarsdottir and D. H. Bovbjerg (1997).

R. B. Lambert and N. K. Lambert (1995).

p. 69   C. A. P. Ruck et al. (1979).

T. Roberts and P. J. Hruby (1997+). Online: http://www.csp.org/chrestomathy

T. Roberts (ed. 2001).

p. 70   Council on Spiritual Practices. www.csp.org

Huston Smith (2001).

R. Forte (ed. 1997).

p. 71   Vallombrosa Conference Center. Owned by the Archdiocese of San Francisco. www.Vallombrosa.org

Institute for Transpersonal Psychology. www.itp.edu

p.72   First Congregational Church of DeKalb — United Church of Christ, 615 North First Street, DeKalb, IL. 815-758-0691.

Chicago Theological Seminary. www.ctschicago.edu

p. 73   United Church of Christ. www.ucc.org

p. 75   L. Grinspoon and J. Bakalar (1979).

p. 76   W. H. Clark (1974). Hallucinogen drug controversy. In: Radouco-Thomas et al.

W. N. Pahnke and W. Richards (1966).

Mysticism Scale: R. W. Hood, Jr. (1995).

Chapter 7: From POTT MUSIC to Spontaneous Remission

p. 80   POTT MUSIC: P.J. Hruby (2001).

p. 82   R. W. Hood (1975).

Journal of Transpersonal Psychology (1969+). Palo Alto, CA: Institute for Transpersonal Psychology.

Council on Spiritual Practices. Thomas B. Roberts. (1997). States of Unitive Consciousness: Research Summary. San Francisco. http://www.csp.org/docs/unitive.html

P. J. Hruby (1966).

D. Lukoff and F. Lu (1988).

p. 84   H. B. Valdimarsdottir and A. A. Stone (1997).

p. 85   M. H. Glock, P. A. Heller, D. Malamud (1992).

A. A. Stone et al. (1987, 1994, 1996).

p. 86   H. B. Valdimarsdottir and A. A. Stone (1997).

R. McCraty et al. (1996).

p. 87   D. McClelland et al. (1982).

D. C. McClelland and A. D. Cheriff (1997).

Timothy Leary (1997).

p. 88   J. B. Jainmott and K. Magloire (1988).

p. 89   *B. O'Regan and C. Hirshberg (1993). Spontaneous Remission*

p. 93   For Pagels see: Diane Rogers (2004).

For Delphic Oracle see: J. R. Hale et al. (2003).

Hamilton College, Clinton, NY. www.hamilton.edu

p. 95   Medical World News (1974). Spontaneous cancer regression – First World Conference asks: How does it work? June 7:13–15.

Y. Ikemi et al. (1975).

C. Weinstock (1983).

A. Meares (1979).

p. 96   W. Richards et al. (1977).

B. Valdimarsdottir and A. A. Stone (1997).

L. Grinspoon and J. Bakalar (1979). *Psychedelic Drugs Reconsidered.*

Chapter 8: Bigger, Stronger, Brighter — A New Relationship with Our Minds

p. 100 Epigraph: William James: (1902/1982).

p. 101 Aldous Huxley's *Doors of Perception* was published in 1954 and had been in print consistently since then in many editions. In current editions *Doors* is printed together with *Heaven and Hell*. I particularly like *Doors* as an example of the kind of trip an educated and sophisticated person can have. In fact, I make it the first reading in my class *Foundations of Psychedelic Studies* both because it was historically a key book because it was the book that alerted many people to the possibilities of psychedelics. However, the word 'psychedelic' hadn't been coined yet. *Doors* also presents thematic ideas the course will consider later in more detail: self-transcendence, Eastern psychologies, sensory intensification, and seeing our minds as restricting what we observe and think (the reducing valve idea). A problem with *Doors* is that this is Aldous Huxley's experience. It portrays his set and setting. Too many people don't realize that if they do mescaline or another psychedelic their set and setting will largely determine their experience. They won't have Huxley's.

Huston Smith's *Cleansing the Doors of Perception* obviously draws its title from Huxley's *Doors*. You'll see I allude to both titles below. *Cleansing* is notable, among other reasons, because Smith is so well known and regarded in the philosophy of religion, and *Cleansing* is both a byproduct of that renown and adds to Smith's stature. When he told me in 1995 that he was to be interviewed by Bill Moyers in a 5-part series on Public Television early in 1996, I invited him to speak at Northern Illinois University. I knew of his long-term interest in the entheogenic use of psychedelics and wanted to schedule him before the TV series made it difficult to do so. In the fall of 1966 he gave 2 speeches at Northern Illinois University. To prepare my students, I collected all of Smith's writings I could find on psychedelics. I realized they would make a fine book, photocopied his articles and sent them to him and via the Council on Spiritual Practices. Smith edited his writings a bit and added introductions. In addition to the trade editions, the Council on Spiritual Practices makes available a deluxe, boxed, limited edition in the style of Wasson's deluxe editions. For information check www.csp.org.

Psychedelic research, review of the literature:

The book that most fully compiles research on psychedelics is Grinspoon and Bakalar's *Psychedelic Drugs Reconsidered* (1997). When I begin to investigate a new topic in psychedelics, *PDR* is usually the first resource I turn to. The 1997 reprint is out of print, and the book deserves another edition. The paperback editions are preferable to the original hardcover edition because of their extensive, topical, annotated bibliography — 40 pages.

Charley Grob's *Hallucinogens* (2002) selects and collects 15 of the best recent articles on hallucinogens (Tarcher/Putnam: New York) and contains appendices on ayahuasca, deconstructing ecstasy, and his analysis of what psychiatrists have learned from psychedelics, or should have learned.

My favorite online broad-scope resource is *The Psychedelic Library*, a rich resource. http://www.psychedelic-library.org. The MAPS website and Heffter website are my favorites for up-to-the minute news: http://www.MAPS.org. and http://www.heffter.org. Both websites accumulate information and are growing in depth every year.

p. 102   Psychedelics as Psychomagnifiers:

Stanislav Grof: In addition to *Realms*, many of his subsequent books describe the amplifying, or magnifying, effect of psychedelics. For example, Grof and Bennett's *The Holotropic Mind* (1992) is a sort of *Realms-lite*. As the name suggests, Grof's *LSD Psychotherapy* (1992) is more for mental health professionals.

Spiritual intelligence: *Psychoactive Sacramentals* (Roberts, 2001) is derived from a conference I helped organize for the Council on Spiritual Practices and the Chicago Theological Seminary. Rather then being a proceedings of the conference, we asked the people who attended to reflect on the conference and write a paper afterwards. *Psych Sacs*'s 25 contributors consider the religious significance of entheogens and the associated questions, problems, and opportunities that they present to contemporary religion.

Robert Forte's anthology *Entheogens and the Future of Religion* preceded *Psych Sacs* in 1997. Now into a second printing, *EFR's* 14 contributors are clergy, scholars, and spiritually interested persons who consider, as the title indicates, entheogens' future role.

Religion and Psychoactive Sacraments: An Entheogen Chrestomathy (www.csp.org/chrestomathy) is my big, multiyear project (1995+). It contains extended bibliographic information and excerpts from over 550 books, dissertations, and topical issues of journals on the topic of entheogens. Customary bibliographic information is given (author, date, title, publisher, and place) as well as

ISBN, a brief description, and contents. Contributors to anthologies are listed, and occasional 'notes' point out items of interest. The excerpts are chosen to present a diversity of ideas about entheogens, some pro, some con, and many making non-judgmental commentary. A search for:

\<mystic or mystical or mysticism> finds over 200 entries
\<consciousness> finds over 199 entries
\<shaman or shamanism> finds over 34 entries
\<LSD> finds over 179 entries
\<peyote> finds over 75 entries
\<ayahuasca> finds over 23 entries
\<science> finds over 91 entries
\<research> finds over 245 entries

By expanding the search to the full Council on Spiritual Practices website, additional resources appear, often in full text. The chrestomathy will continue to grow as new entries are added from time to time. *Religion and Psychoactive Sacraments: An Entheogen Chrestomathy* is published online as a free service of the Council on Spiritual Practices.

Psychedelic Psychotherapy: In addition to Grof's books listed above and Grinspoon and Bakalar, my favorite source of information on psychedelic psychotherapy up to 1995 is *Psycholytic and Psychedelic Therapy Research 1931–1995: A Complete International Bibliography* by Torsten Passie (1997). Passie lists 687 studies as well as conferences and main bibliographic sources. Studies are cross listed by diagnostic category, types of patients, drug used, and author. This is an enormous contribution to the field.

General psychedelic resource, MAPS' website: For keeping up to date on current research, I use the *MAPS Bulletin* (Multidisciplinary Association for Psychedelic Studies) in addition to the standard medical and mental health resources: http://www.maps.org. This is one rich website! As you've probably guessed, I assign my *Foundations of Psychedelic Studies* class to explore around it, and they always find hidden treasures.

p. 105 The Singlestate Fallacy: An earlier presentation of the singlestate fallacy with an emphasis on how it applies to religious studies is in my chapter 'An Entheogen Idea-Map — Future Explorations' in *Psychoactive Sacramentals: Essays on Entheogens and Religion* published in 2001 by the Council on Spiritual Practices.

p. 106 Meditation research: For examples see Murphy, Donovan, and Taylor (1997). From neurophysiological and health-related studies to psychological and religious ones, the constantly growing field of meditation research illustrates the range of topics that a mindbody research paradigm can encompass. See *Consilience* for an extension of this idea.

p. 107 MDMA and serotonin reuptake: *The Economist*, Pharmacogenomics: The Agony and the Ecstasy. March 10, 2005.

p. 108 *The Economist*, Pharmacogenomics: The Agony and the Ecstasy. March 10, 2005.

p. 110 A Comparison of Singlestate and Multistate Paradigms: General Assumptions: table adapted from Roberts (1989).

Chapter 9: The Multistate Paradigm

p. 113 Wider perspective, related mindbody topics: As I present multistate theory presented in this book, it is focused primarily on the multistate nature of our minds and on multistate education (especially Chapters 13 and 14 in this book). For a broader multistate perspective, see Roberts (1989). Near the end of that article, 4 tables contrast how singlestate approaches and multistate approaches consider various concepts: 'A Comparison of Single-state Psychologies and Mindbody Multistate Psychologies.' Table 1 is General Intellectual Paradigm: Table 2, Major Psychologies: Table 3: Cognition and Learning: and Table 4: Mental Health.

'Mindbody' vs. 'Consciousness': Most importantly, the word *mindbody* explicitly expresses what I mean. I am considering our minds and our bodies as one united thing (*mindbody*) and how this combination varies from one moment to the next (*mindbody states*). And I am writing about all the different ways this combination, or recipe, can change — about various mindbody states. *Consciousness* is a fine word, but in my experience it has so many different meanings that when people say *consciousness* it sounds at first as if they're talking about the same thing, but really they are using different meanings and talking about different things. For example, *consciousness* can simply mean not being asleep, in a coma, or unconscious. It can mean aware of one's surroundings or responding to one's environment. It can mean the thoughts or feelings someone has because of his or her social location in society as in 'women's consciousness' or 'proletarian consciousness.' Another synonym is 'psychophysiological state': see Green, Green, and Walters (1970). Sometimes *consciousness* can indicate level of spiritual awareness or growth as in 'moving to a higher level of consciousness.' It might also mean whatever happens to be on one's mind; years ago I saw a sign by the sink at the Institute of Transpersonal Psychology: 'Have cleanliness consciousness. Please wash your cups after you use them.' There's nothing the matter with any of these uses of the word *consciousness*, but they lend themselves to being easily misinterpreted. So in hopes of being clear that I am writing about a unified, combined state of mind and body considered as one, I opt for *mindbody* and *mindbody state*.

p. 114 Tart's subsystems: These are listed and briefly described in a table 'Experiential Criteria for Detecting an Altered State of Consciousness' on pages 12–13 of Tart (1975). Here and in the 'Wild Parameters' section below, I'm using Tart's 10 plus my 2 additions— 'moral sense' and 'intuition'— not just as ways of detecting a shift in mindbody state, but also as those states' psychological ingredients.

This list from Tart's *States of Consciousness* along with Benny Shanon's list of psychological parameters from *Antipodes of the Mind*, may be useful nominees for a more complete list of parameters that researchers should consider when examining mindbody states. They each, of course, can be used as independent and/or dependent variables for future multistate experiments.

p. 115 Compositions for mind in infinite variations: From Roberts (1981).

p. 116 Mindbody Psychotechnologies: William James (1902/1982).

p. 117 Charles Tart (1969), reprinted several times in paperback.

Theodore X. Barber (ed. 1976).

Ernest Rossi (1993).

Michael Murphy (1992).

American Psychological Association: Cardena, Lynn, and Krippner (ed. 2002); Imants Baruss (2003).

Chapter 10: Intelligence, Creativity, Metaintelligence

p. 120 Howard Gardner (1983).

p. 121 Dream problem solving and creativity: All the examples of solving problems in dreams are from MacKenzie (1965).

Psychedelic problem solving: Frank Barron, 'The Creative Process and the Psychedelic Experience' http://www.psychedelic-library.org/barron.htm.

Willis W Harman, Robert H. McKim, Robert E. Mogar, James Fadiman, and Myron Stolaroff (1966). This is easier to find as Chapter 30 in Tart (1969).

p. 123 Kary Mullis: Quoted in Doblin (1994). For more information see Mullis (1998).

p. 124 Francis Crick: Rees (2004). The connection between Crick and early LSD personages is supported in Tendler & May (1984), Chapter 13, 'The Badlands — Brotherhood International' (page 178)

Serotonin Club: www.serotoninclub.org The Serotonin Club is an international association for biomedical scientists who are interested in any aspect of research on serotonin (5-hydroxytryptamine). It was founded over 10 years ago and currently has a membership of around 450 persons worldwide. Members receive a regular newsletter with information on scientific meetings, news of members and any other matters of interest to those working on serotonin.

The Club sponsors a satellite meeting to the International Congress of Pharmacology (IUPHAR) Congress every 4 years and occasional other meetings. It also gives financial support to assist young scientists to attend these meetings. The Club also hosts annual lectures and dinners which are held in association with the American Society for Neuroscience meeting and one of the meetings of the British Pharmacological Society (usually the Winter meeting).

p. 125 David E. Nichols (1999–2000):

'LET ME START OFF by suggesting that a significant number of the people in this room tonight and indeed a significant percentage of serotonin researchers worldwide first gained their interest in serotonin through some association with psychedelic agents. For some people it may have been as a participant in a legitimate scientific clinical experiment, others may have done some personal experimentation during the 1960s. Perhaps others read some of the rich and interesting literature describing the powerful effect on the psyche of these drugs and developed an academic curiosity, or perhaps still others developed an interest through the drug abuse aspect, 'Why do people enjoy taking these drugs?' Whatever the motivation, I would still assert that a significant percentage of the serotonin researchers in the world today developed their research focus through some connection to psychedelic drugs.'
http://www.maps.org/news-letters/v09n04/0945nicALT.

html If this link doesn't work (as it didn't for me), go to the MAPS website and search the title.

MAPS Bulletin: The 'creativity issue' — Vol. X, No. 3, 2000 — is a good source of addition instances of psychedelic-assisted creativity. I assign it in my *Foundations of Psychedelic Studies* class as the main reading in creativity.

p. 126 Shareware: Bob Wallace (1997). Wallace goes on to say, 'I think psychedelics help you in general go beyond the normal way of doing things, and you really open your mind to more possibilities that maybe seem obvious in retrospect but you'd never think of if you were going along the normal way of doing things.' This program shows Mullis receiving the Noble Prize and interviews him about the role of psychedelics in his discovery.

p. 127 A Comparison of Singlestate and Multistate Paradigms: Cognition: table adapted from Roberts (1989).

p. 128 Sternberg, Robert J. (1988).

Chapter 11: Psychology, Science, and Survival

p. 135 Michael Winkelman (2000).

Society for the Anthropology of Consciousness: The SAC holds regular meetings and publishes the journal *Anthropology of Consciousness*. http://sunny.moorpark.cc.ca.us/~baker/sac/home.html.

p. 136 The Divine Other: Roberts, Thomas. B. (book manuscript under construction) *Increasing Spiritual Intelligence: Chemical Input, Religious Output*.

Roberts, Thomas B. (2006).

Roberts, Thomas B. (2004). Combined book review of Newberg et al. (2001), in which the authors studied areas of brain activity and inactivity during meditation in Franciscan nuns and Tibetan meditators, and Fuller (2000). I made the obvious multistate suggestion that *Why God's* authors should use their instrumentation to study the combined brain effects and subjective effects that Fuller writes about.

Roberts, Thomas B. (2003b). Triple book review of Strassman (2001), Jansen (2001), and Saunders et al. (2000).

Roberts, Thomas B. (2003a). Book review of Shanon (2003c).

Roberts, Thomas B. (editor 2001).

Roberts, Thomas B. & Hruby, Paula. J. (Compilers 1992–2002). Over 550 entries averaging about 3 single-spaced pages each. So far as I know, this is the world's major reference on entheogen books, dissertations, and topic issues of journals. Available: http://www.csp.org/chrestomathy/

p. 137 Benny Shanon (2002).

p. 139 Stanislav Grof (1975). *Realms* is my nominee as one of the great books. Nothing is so central to our view of human nature as our ideas about our minds, and *Realms* presents a new, more inclusive map as well as the psychedelic method of exploring the human mind. I expect *Realms* to become recognized as a key book in intellectual history. Of course, I use it in my *Foundations of Psychedelic Studies* class.

p. 140 A Comparison of Singlestate and Multistate Paradigms: Psychologies: table adapted from Roberts (1989).

Abraham H. Maslow: Self-actualization is mistakenly considered the top of Maslow's needs-hierarchy of motivation. Between 1962 and 1968, he divided self-actualizers into transcenders and non-transcenders and added self-transcendence as a stage above self-actualization. This is marked by his prefaces to the first and second editions of his book *Toward a Psychology of Being* as well as in other writings. For details see: Roberts. (1978). See also: Maslow. (1967), (1968). The Preface to the Second edition of *Toward a Psychology of Being* (1968) marks Maslow's transition from seeing self-actualization as the top of his need hierarchy to seeing self-transcendence as the top.

p. 142 Broader Databases: Lester Grinspoon and James Bakalar (1979). The Whitehead quotation is on page vii.

p. 143 Charles Tart (1969). The book as been reprinted several times in paperback editions.

p. 144 Myron Stolaroff: (1994). *Thanatos to Eros: Thirty-five Years of Psychedelic Exploration*. Berlin: Verlag fur Wissenschaft und Bildung. Pages 41–43.

p. 145 Myron Stolaroff: (1999). Are Psychedelics Useful in the Practice of Buddhism? *Journal of Humanistic Psychology*. Vol. 39, No. 1, pages 60 – 80.

Buddhism: A topical issue 'Buddhism and Psychedelics' of *Tricycle: The Buddhist Review* (Vol. 4, No. 1, Fall 1996) presents 14 articles on this topic. Some are pro, others con, and some do not judge. Most of the pro articles take a qualified stand, warning users not to become attached to psychedelics or the experiences they promote.

Charles Tart: (1991).

Roger Walsh: 1983. Excerpt from page 117.

p. 147 Adaptive Advantage: Stephen J. Gould (1996).

Psychedelic Science: Originally shown on BBC TV in 1998, and more recently on America's A&E channel, I show this videotape to my *Foundations of Psychedelic Studies* class during the 1st or 2nd week of class. It's an excellent introduction to psychedelics' history and an update on more recent developments.

Chapter 12: The Major Intellectual Opportunity of Our Times — the Central Multistate Question

p. 151 Lawrence S. Kubie (1954).

p. 154 Benny Shanon (2002).

p. 155 *Consilience*: Edward Wilson (1998).

biochemistry: Daniel M. Perrine. (1996). *The Chemistry of Mind-Altering Drugs* was chosen as one of only two books in the field of chemistry to be honored by the Association of American Publishers in their 'Best of 1996' Awards. Additionally, it has been selected by CHOICE as one of the 'Outstanding Academic Books reviewed in 1997.'

Greek mythology: Carl A. P. Ruck, Blaise Staples, and Clark Heinrich (2001).

Biblical history: Carl A. P. Ruck (2003). Available online: http://www.thehempire.com/pm/comments/281_0_1_0_ C/. A google.com search will turn up lots more sites that contain this.

p. 156 Psychead: A project yet to be accomplished.

Chapter 13: It Means Something Different to be Well Educated

p. 162 Epigraph: Roger Walsh (1983).

p. 164 All the Questions Get Reasked: see Roberts (1981).

Churches and Increasing Spiritual Intelligence: Roberts (2006).

Trail to Discovering Topics: Roberts (1998).

p. 166 Kenneth W. Tupper (2002, 2003).

p. 167   A Comparison of Singlestate and Multistate Paradigms: Learning. This table and the 4 other similar tables are adapted from Roberts (1989).

p. 168   'Chemical Input, Religious Output': See note under p. 194

Chapter 14: Enlarging Learning

p. 172   Epigraph: Peter C. Whybrow (2005).

p. 173   Enlarging educational possibilities: Thomas B. Roberts (1985, March-April; 2003).

New books, articles, and websites are frequently published on these topics. Here are some of my favorites, with a special emphasis on schools.

Biofeedback: With its empirical observations grounded in measurements of physiological changes in our bodies, for may people biofeedback opened the door to recognizing (1) that our bodies can produce measurable biological changes, (2) that some of these accompany and document significant alterations in states of consciousness ('mindbody states'), (3) that higher level cognitive processes such as thoughts and visual images can influence these bodily shifts, and (4) that we can learn the cognitive processes that influence our bodies with our minds. Numbers 3 and 4 are especially important because they show that influences go 'downward' from mind-to-body as well as 'upward' from body-to-mind. It's a two-way street. The two major control systems in our bodies are the nervous system and the endocrine (hormonal) system. We can learn to take many aspects of these into control, and various mindbody techniques assist in learning this. This impresses me as the ultimate physical education of the future — discovering what the fullest extent of bodily control is, then learning to do this. A websearch for *biofeedback* plus the application you are looking for will usually bring up many Internet sites and pages.

Meditation: Murdock (1987), Murphy et al. (1997).

Imagery in Sports: Murphy (1992).

Imagery in Teaching: Wass (2000).

Imagery and the Placebo Effect: Harrington (editor, 1997).

Hypnosis: Hilgard (1977), Rossi (1993).

Dreams: Krippner et al. (2003).

For an earlier discussion of this, see: Roberts (1981a).

p. 174 Anomalies: Grinspoon and Bakalar. (1979). Grof's books on psychedelic psychotherapy have enough challenges to keep people scratching their heads of decades (at least): Grof (1975), Grof and Bennett (1992). Most books on psychedelics contain their modicum of anomalies. People who have tolerance for ambiguity will thrive in psychedelic research (and multistate research in general); those who feel comfortable with a low tolerance for ambiguity had best stick to singlestate research.

Collections: Cardena et al. (editors) (2002). Charles Tart's *Altered States of Consciousness* (1969) is the key book that organized the study of other states of consciousness into one field when it collected research on various mindbody psychotechnologies into one volume.

Kuhn (1962). This is the book that made 'paradigm' famous and gave a rationale to anyone working in any odd field: 'I'm starting a new paradigm.' Mea culpa, too.

p. 175 Princeton Engineering Anomalies Research: Jahn and Dunne. (1988). The 8 characteristic conditions or situations (set and setting) are listed in Nelson et al. (1998). Try poking around here: http://www.princeton.edu/~pear/ for some hot anomalies.

p. 177 Set and setting: These, plus the psychoactive drug and its dose, are the 3 major influences on the experiences people have with psychoactives. The oldest use of 'set and setting' that I've been able to trace was in Leary et al. (1963): 'The role of various set and setting variables was described and a tentative psychological mechanism proposed to account for the effects of these variables.' (page 572)

Parapsychological abilities related to mindbody states: Eysenck and Sargent (1982).

p. 178 A Comparison of Singlestate and Multistate Paradigms: Mental Health: table adapted from Roberts (1989).

p. 181 The God Within: Roberts (2006).

p. 182 Transpersonal examples abound — here are some:

International Journal of Transpersonal Studies. (1997+). Honolulu: Panigada Press.

Journal of Transpersonal Psychology. (1969+). Stanford, CA: Transpersonal Institute.

Maslow (1967, 1968).

Roberts (1978).

Walsh and Vaughan (1993).

Aldous Huxley: *The Doors of Perception.* (1954 and many other editions). *Entheogens – Sacramentals or Sacrilege?* http://www.cedu.niu.edu/epf/edpsych/faculty/roberts/index_roberts.html

Intellectual adventures: Roberts & Hruby (1992-2002) contains excerpts and extended bibliographic information from over 550 books and dissertations. http://www.csp.org/chrestomathy

'Chemical Input, Religious Output': See note under p. 194

p. 183   Strassman (2001).

Shanon (2002).

p. 184   Sasha and Ann Shulgin (1991, 1997).

p. 185   Anthropology: Bourguignon, (1973).

Paradigm: I'm jumping the hopeful gun here. In his 1962 paradigm-establishing book *The Structure of Scientific Revolutions*, Kuhn describes a paradigm as a model that is followed by a group of scientists as a basis for their scientific efforts and gives an overall orientation to their work. Actually, I am proposing the multistate model as a paradigm, but it doesn't qualify as a paradigm because it doesn't ('yet' I like to think) have a group of followers. I think the multistate model qualifies as a potentially rich paradigm because it includes such things as assumptions about what is real, theories, concepts, the nature of legitimate questions and their answers, research methods and instruments, and prototype examples of research.

p. 188   Rudgley (1993).

Chapter 15: Is the Reprogrammable Brain Adaptigenic?

p. 191   Multidisciplinary Association for Psychedelic Studies: www.maps.org

p. 192   Sartre: Riedlinger (1982).

Grof (1977).

p. 193   centering: Hendricks and Wills (1975). Hendricks and Roberts (1977). Murdock (1987).

p. 194   Increasing Spiritual Intelligence: Roberts (2006). I am expanding this chapter into a book manuscript tentatively titled *Increasing Spiritual Intelligence: Chemical Input, Religious Output* (manuscript in preparation).

Hofmann quotation: From an interview with Albert Hofmann, in Chapter 2 of Walsh and Grob (Editors) (2005). A really fine book.

p. 195   Neuroplasticity: Schwartz and Begley. (2002). Sometimes these ideas and related ones are called 'cellular plasticity' or 'cerebral plasticity.'

p. 198   Bioethics: Guterman (2004), Gazzaniga (2005), Naam (2005).

p. 199   Value shift from mystical experiences: Miller and C' de Baca (2001), Learner and Lyvers (2004).

Michael Harner quotation: Interview with Michael Harner in Chapter 9 of Walsh and Grob (2005).

Center for Cognitive Liberty and Ethics, www.cognitiveliberty.org

p. 201   Community Psychedelic Centers, Inc. — Prospectus for an IPO: Thomas B. Roberts (unpublished manuscript). DeKalb, IL: Northern Illinois University.

p. 202   G. W. Pharmaceutical: www.gwpharm.com. Possible conflict of interest statement: I am a shareholder in GWP.

p. 205   Wulff quotation: (1991), page 639.

Bibliography

Barber, Theodore X. (editor) (1976). *Advances in Altered States of Consciousness and Human Potentialities*. New York: Psychological Dimensions.

Barron, Frank. "The Creative Process and the Psychedelic Experience." http://www.psychedelic-library.org/barron.htm.

Baruss, Imants (2003). *Alterations of Consciousness*. Washington, DC.

Bishop, Peter (1981). *Archetypal Topology*. Spring Pub., Zurich.

Bourguignon, Erika (1973). *Religion, Altered States of Consciousness, and Social Change*. Columbus, OH: Ohio University Press.

Bugental, J. F. T. (Ed.) 1967. *Challenges of Humanistic Psychology*, New York: McGraw Hill.

Campbell, Joseph (1949). *The Hero with a Thousand Faces*. (Bollingen Series) Princeton, NJ: Princeton University Press. Available in other editions too.

Campbell, Joseph (1982). *Myths to Live By*. New York: Bantam. (Arkana reprint edition, 1993).

Cardena, Etzel, Stephen Jay Lynn, and Stanley Krippner (editors). (2002). *Varieties of Anomalous Experience: Examining the Scientific Evidence*. Washington, DC: American Psychological Association.

Clark, W. H. (1974). Hallucinogen drug controversy. In: S. Radouco-Thomas, A. Villeneuve, C. Radouco-Thomas. (eds.) *Pharmacologie, toxicologie, et abuse de psychotomimétiques (hallucinogènes) [Pharmacology, Toxicology, and Abuse of Psychomimetics (Hallucinogens)]*. Quebec Les Presses l'Université Laval. Pages 411–418.

Cott, Jonathan: (1973). *Notes on Fairy Faith and the Ideas of Childhood in Beyond the Looking Glass*. New York: Stonehill Pub.

Doblin, Rick. (1994). Laying the Groundwork. *Newsletter of the Multidisciplinary Association for Psychedelic Studies*, Vol. 4, No. 4, Spring. http://65.18.176.18/news-letters/v04n4/04401lay.html.

Eysenck, Hans J. and Sargent, Carl (1982). *Explaining the Unexplained: Mysteries of the Paranormal*. London: Weidenfeld and Nicholson.

Farrell, Barry (1966). Scientists, Theologians, Mystics, Swept Up in a Psychic Revolution. *LIFE*, March 25, page 30.

Forte, R. (ed.) (1997). *Entheogens and the Future of Religion*. San Francisco: Council on Spiritual Practices.

Freedman, Daniel X. (1968). On the Use and Abuse of LSD. *Archives of General Psychiatry*, Vol. 18, pages 330-347.

Fuller, Robert C. (2000). *Stairways to Heaven: Drugs in American Religious History*. Boulder, CO: Westview Press.

Gardner, Howard (1983). *Frames of Mind: The Theory of Multiple Intelligences*. New York: Basic Books.

Gazzaniga, Michael S. (2005). *The Ethical Brain*. New York: Dana Press.

Glock, M. H., P. A. Heller, D. Malamud. (1992). *Saliva as a Diagnostic Fluid: January 1982 through April 1992*. Bethesda, MD: National Library of Medicine, National Institutes of Health.

Gould, Stephen J. (1996). *Full House: The Spread of Excellence from Plato to Darwin*. New York: Harmony Books.

Graves, Robert (1948). *The White Goddess*. New York: McGraw-Hill. Graves speaks of the 'German folk-story Snow White' on p. 348.

Green, Elmer, Alyse Green, and Dale Walters (1970). Voluntary control of internal states: Psychological and physiological. *Journal of Transpersonal Psychology*, Vol. 2, No. 1, pages 1-26.

Grinspoon, L. and J. Bakalar. (1979). *Psychedelic Drugs Reconsidered*. New York: Bantam Books. (Reprint edition 1997 by Lindesmith Center, New York).

Grinspoon, Lester and James B. Bakalar (ed.) (1983). *Psychedelic Reflections*. New York: Human Sciences Press.

Grob, Charley *Hallucinogens: A Reader* (2002) (Tarcher/Putnam: New York)

Grof, Stanislav (1975). *Realms of the Human Unconscious: Observations from LSD Psychotherapy*. New York: E. P. Dutton & Co. This was reprinted in 1976 in paperback edition. Condor Books, Souvenir Press (E & A) reprinted *Realms* in a paperback edition in 1993. Grof refines and recapitulates his map of our minds in several of his subsequent books.

Grof, Stanislav (1977). The Perinatal Roots of Wars, Totalitarianism, and Revolutions: Observations from LSD Research. *Journal of Psychohistory*, Vol. 4 (winter), No. 3 pages 269–308.

Grof, Stanislav (1980). *LSD Psychotherapy*. Hunter House, Pomona, CA. (Republished in 1992 in a 2nd edition by Hunter House in Alameda CA. Several other editions exist.)

Grof, Stanislav and Hal Z. Bennett (1992). *The Holotropic Mind: The Three Levels of Human Consciousness and How They Shape our Lives*. San Francisco, CA: HarperCollins.

Guterman, Lila (2004). Gray Matters. *Chronicle of Higher Education*. Vol. 1, pages 113-117.

Hale, J. R., J. Z. de Boer, J. P. Chanton and H. A. Spiller (2003, August). Questioning the Delphic Oracle. *Scientific American*, August, pages 66–73.

Harman, Willis W, Robert H. McKim, Robert E. Mogar, James Fadiman, and Myron Stolaroff (1966). Psychedelic Agents in Creative Problem Solving: A Pilot Study. *Psychological Reports*, Vol. 19, pages 211–227.

Harrington, Anne (editor) (1997). *The Placebo Effect: An Interdisciplinary Exploration.* Cambridge, MA: Harvard University Press.

Hayes, Charles. (editor) (2000). *Tripping: An Anthology of True-life Psychedelic Adventures.* New York: Penguin.

Hendricks, Gay and Russel Wills (1975). *The Centering Book: Awareness Activities for Children, Parents and Teachers.* Englewood Cliffs, NJ: Prentice-Hall.

Hendricks, Gay and Thomas B. Roberts (1977). *The Second Centering Book: More Awareness Activities for Children, Parent, and Teachers.* Englewood Cliffs, NJ: Prentice-Hall.

Hilgard, Ernest (1977). *Divided Consciousness: Multiple Controls in Human Thought and Action.* New York: Wiley.

Hillman, James (1974, Spring). Anima II Spring Publ, Zurich.

Hillman, James (1977, Spring). *An Inquiry into Image.* Zurich: Spring Pub.

Holland, Julie (editor) (2001). *Ecstasy: The Complete Guide: A Comprehensive Look at the Risks and Benefits of MDMA.* Rochester, VT: Inner Traditions.

Hofmann, Albert (1980). *LSD: My Problem Child: Reflections on Sacred Drugs, Mysticism, and Science.* Translated by Jonathan Ott. New York: McGraw-Hill.

Hood, R. W. (1975). The construction and preliminary validation of a measure of reported mystical experience. *Journal for the Scientific Study of Religion,* Vol. 14, No. 1, pages 29–41.

Hood, R. W. Jr. (1995). The facilitation of religious experience. In R. W. Hood, Jr. (ed.) *Handbook of Religious Experience.* Birmingham, AL: Religious Education Press.

Horgan, John (2003). *Rational Mysticism : Spirituality Meets Science in the Search for Enlightenment.* Howard Miflin.

Hruby, P. J. (1966). *The Varieties of Mystical Experience, Spiritual Practices, and Psychedelic Drug Use Among College Students.* DeKalb, IL: Northern Illinois University (Unpublished doctoral dissertation).

Hruby, P.J. (2001). Unitive Consciousness and Pahnke's Good Friday Experiment. Chapter 6, pages 59–68 in Roberts (2001).

Huxley, Aldous (1954), *Doors of Perception.* New York: Harper and Row.

Ikemi, Y., S. Nakagawa, T. Nakagawa and S. Mineyasu (1975). Psychosomatic consideration of cancer patients who have made a narrow escape from death. *Dynamiche Psychiatry,* Vol. 31, pages 77–92.

Jahn, Robert and Dunne, Brenda (1988). *Margins of Reality: The Role of Consciousness in the Physical World.* New York: Wiley

Jainmott, J. B. and K. Magloire (1988). Academic stress, social support, and secretory Iummunoglobulin A. *Journal of Personality and Social Psychology,* Vol. 55, pages 803–810.

James, William (1982). *The Varieties of Religious Experience: A Study in Human Nature.* New York: Penguin Books. (Original work published in 1902)

Jansen, Karl (2001). *Ketamine: Dreams and Realities*. Sarasota, FL: Multi-disciplinary Association for Psychedelic Studies.

Jung, C. G. (1966). *The Spirit in Man, Art and Literature*. Princeton: Bollingen.

Jung, C. G. (1973). *Four Archetypes*. Princeton: Bollingen,. The chapter 'The Phenomenology of the Spirit in Fairytales' is especially relevant.

Jung, C. G. (1976). *The Vision Seminars*. Zurich: Spring Publications. Several excellent accounts of fairy tale symbology.

Krippner, Stanley and Achterberg, Jeanne (2000). Anomalous Healing Experiences. Chapter 11, pages 353–395 in Cardena et al. (2000).

Kubie, Lawrence S. (1954). The Forgotten Man of Education. *Harvard Alumni Bulletin*, Vol. 56, pages 349-353.

Kuhn, Thomas S. (1962). *The Structure of Scientific Revolutions*. Chicago: The University of Chicago Press.

Lambert, R. B. and N. K. Lambert (1995). The effects of humor on secretory immunoglobulin levels in school-aged children. *Pediatric Nursing*, Vol. 21, No. 1 (Jan–Feb), pages 16–19, 28–29.

Learner, Michael and Michael Lyvers (2004). Cross-cultural comparison of values, beliefs, and sense of coherence in psychedelic drug users. *Bulletin of the Multidisciplinary Association for Psychedelic Studies*. Vol. 14, No. 1, pages 9–10.

Leary, Timothy, George H. Levine, and Ralph Metzner (1963). 'Reactions to Psilocybin Administered in a Supportive Environment', *The Journal of Nervous and Mental Disease*, Vol. 137, No. 6, pages 561–573.

Leary, Timothy (1997). *Flashbacks*. Los Angeles, CA: Tarcher.

Lukoff, D. and F. Lu (1988). Transpersonal psychology research review. Topic Mystical Experiences. *Journal of Transpersonal Psychology*, Vol. 20, No. 2, pages 161–184.

Lyttle, Tom (1994). *Psychedelic Essays*. New York: Barricade Books.

MacKenzie, Norman (1965). *Dreams and Dreaming*. New York: Vanguard. This book contains the information on Stevenson, Condorcet, Blake, Kekule, and Hilprecht.

Markoff, John (2005). *What the Dormouse Said: How the 60s Counterculture Shaped the Personal Computer Industry*. New York: Viking.

Maslow, Abraham H. (1967). Self-actualization and Beyond. In Bugental 1967 (pp. 279-286).

Maslow, Abraham H. (1968). *Toward a Psychology of Being*. Princeton: D. Van Nostrand. (Second edition).

McClelland, D. C. and A. D. Cheriff (1997). Iminunoenhancing effects of humor on secretory IgA and resistance to respiratory infections. *Psychology and Health*, Vol. 12, pages 329–344.

McClelland, D., C. Alexander, and E. Marks. (1982). The need for power, stress, immune function, and illness among male prisoners. *Journal of Abnormal Psychology*, Vol. 91, pages 61–70.

McCraty, R., M. Atkinson, G. Rein, and A. D. Watkins. (1996). Music enhances the effect of positive emotional states on salivary IgA. *Stress Medicine*, Vol. 12, No. 3, pages 167–175.

McNamara, Patrick (editor). (2006). *The Psychology of Religious Experience.* Vol. III in the 3-vol. set *Religion and Brain*. Westport, CT: Praeger/ Greenwood Publishers.

Meares, A. (1979). Regression of cancer of the rectum after intensive meditation. *Medical Journal of Australia*, Vol. 2 (Nov. 17), pages 539–540.

Medical World News (1974). Spontaneous cancer regression — First World Conference asks: How does it work? June 7, pages 13–15.

Miller, William R. and Janet C'de Baca (2001). *Quantum Change: When Epiphanies and Sudden Insights Transform Ordinary Lives.* New York: Guilford Press.

Mullis, Kary (1998). *Dancing Naked in the Mind Field.* New York: Pantheon Autobiography.

Murdock, Maureen (1987). *Spinning Inward: Using Guided Imagery with Children for Learning, Creativity & Relaxation.* Boston, MA: Shambala.

Murphy, Michael, Steven Donovan, and Eugene Taylor (1997). *The Physical and Psychological Effects of Meditation: A Review of Contemporary Research With a Comprehensive Bibliography, 1931–1996.* Petaluma, CA: Institute of Noetic Sciences.

Murphy, Michael: (1992). *The Future of the Body: Explorations Into the Further Evolution of Human Nature.* Los Angeles, CA: J. P. Tarcher.

Myers, Isabel Briggs and Katherine Cook Briggs (1998). *Myers-Briggs Type Indicator.* Distributed by Center for Applied Psychological Type, Gainesville, FL.

Naam, Ramez (2005). *More than Human: Embracing the Promise of Biological Enhancement.* New York: Broadway.

Nelson, R. D. Jahn, R. G., Dunne, B. J., Dobyns, Y. H. and Bradish, G. J. (1998). 'FieldREG II: Consciousness Field Effects: Replications and Explorations,' *Journal of Scientific Exploration*, Vol. 12, No. 3, pages 425–454.

Newberg, Andrew, Eugene D'Aquili, and Vince Rause. (2001). *Why God Won't Go Away: Brain Science and the Biology of Belief.* New York: Ballantine Books.

Nichols, David E. (1999-2000). From Eleusis to PET Scans: The Mysteries of Psychedelics. *MAPS Bulletin*, Vol. 9, No. 4, pages 50-55. Edited address to the Serotonin Club, held at the Annual Meeting of the Society for Neuroscience.

O'Regan, B. and C. Hirshberg (1993). *Spontaneous Remission: An Annotated Bibliography.* Sausalito, CA: Institute of Noetic Sciences.

Pahnke, W. N. and W. Richards. (1966). Implications of LSD and experimental mysticism. *Journal of Religion & Health*, Vol. 5, pages 175–208. (Reprinted in: C. T. Tart (1969). *Altered States of Consciousness: A Book of Readings.* New York: John Wiley)

Pascal, Jeremy (1981). *Fifty Years of the Movies.* New York: Hamlyn.

Passie, T. (1997). *Psycholytic and Psychedelic Therapy Research 1931–1995: A Complete International Bibliography*. Hanover, Germany: Laurentius Publishers.

Perrine, Daniel M. (1996). *The Chemistry of Mind-Altering Drugs: History, Pharmacology, and Cultural Context*. Washington, DC: American Chemical Society. Republished by Oxford University Press.

Rees, Alun (2004) . 'Nobel Prize genius Crick was high on LSD when he discovered the secret of life.' *Mail on Sunday* (London) August 8, Section FB, pages 44–45. Available online:
    http://web.lexisnexis.com/universe/document? ...

Richards, W., J. Rhead, F. DiLeo, R. Yensen and A. Kurland. (1977). The peak experience variable in DPT-assisted psychotherapy with cancer patients. *Journal of Psychedelic Drugs* 9(1): 1–10.

Riedlinger, (1982). Sartre's Rite of Passage. *Journal of Transpersonal Psychology*. Vol. 14, No. 2, pages 105–123.

Roberts, Thomas B. (1978). Beyond Self-actualization. *ReVision: The Journal of Consciousness and Change,* Vol. 1, No. 1, pages 42–45.

Roberts, Thomas B. (1981) New Learning: Consciousness, Psychology, and Education. *Phoenix: Journal of Transpersonal Anthropology*, Vol. 5, No. 1, pages 79–116.

Roberts, Thomas B. (1985, March-April). States of consciousness: A new intellectual direction, a new teacher education direction. *Journal of Teacher Education* Vol. 36, No.2, pages 55–58.

Roberts, Thomas B. (1986). *Brainstorm*: A Psychological Odyssey. *Journal of Humanistic Psychology*, Vol. 26, No. 1, pages 126–136.

Roberts, Thomas B. (1987). Is There a Placebo Ability? *Advances: Journal of the Institute for the Advancement of Health*. Vol. 4, No. 1, page 5. (letter to the editor).

Roberts, Thomas B. (1989) Multistate Education: Metacognitive Implications of the Mindbody Psychotechnologies. *Journal of Transpersonal Psychology*, Vol. 21, No. 1, pages 83–102.

Roberts, Thomas B., and Paula Jo Hruby (1992–2001). *Religion and Psychoactive Sacraments: An Entheogen Chrestomathy*
    http://www.csp.org/chrestomathy

Roberts, Thomas B. (1995). States of Unitive Consciousness: Research Summary. Council on Spiritual Practices: San Francisco.
    http://www.csp.org/docs/unitive.htm1.

Roberts, Thomas B. (1998). Multidisciplinary approaches to psychedelic studies. *MAPS Bulletin*, Vol. VII, No. 1, pages 38–41.
    http://www.maps.org/news-letters/v08n1/083138rob.html.

Roberts, Thomas B. (1999). Do entheogen-induced mystical experiences boost the immune system? Psychedelics, peak experiences, and wellness. *Advances in Mind-Body Medicine*. Vol. 15, No. 2, pages 139–147.

Roberts, Thomas B. (editor) (2001). *Psychoactive Sacramentals: Essays on Entheogens and Religion*. San Francisco: Council on Spiritual Practices.

Roberts, Thomas B. (2003a). A New Relationship with our Minds —
Multistate Mind. *Thresholds in Education*, Vol. 29, No. 3, pp. 36–40.

Roberts, Thomas B. (2003b). Book review of Rick Strassman's *DMT: The
Spirit Molecule: A Doctor's Revolutionary Research into the Biology of
Near-Death and Mystical Experiences of Karl Jansen's, Ketamine: Dreams
and Realities*, and of Nicholas Saunders, Anja Nicholas, and Michelle
Pauli's *In Search of the Ultimate High: Spiritual Experience Through
Psychoactives*. Reviewed in *International Journal for the Psychology of
Religion*. Vol. 13, No.1, pages 75–77.

Roberts, Thomas B. (2003c). Book review of Benny Shanon's *The Antipodes of the Mind: Charting the Phenomenology of the Ayahuasca Experience*.
Reviewed in *Anthropology of Consciousness*, Vol. 14, No. 1, pages 75–79.

Roberts, Thomas B. (2004) Book review of Andrew Newberg, Eugene
D'Aquili, and Vince Rause's *Why God Won't Go Away: Brain Science
and the Biology of Belief* and of Robert C. Fuller's *Stairways to Heaven:
Drugs in American Religious History*. Reviewed in *International Journal
for the Psychology of Religion* Vol. 14, No. 2, pages 139–145.

Roberts, Thomas B. (2006). Chemical Input, Religious Output—
Entheogens: A Pharmatheology Sampler. Chapter in Volume III, *Psy-
chology of Religious Experience*, of a 3-volume set edited by Patrick
McNamara, Ph.D., MD, (Boston University Medical School.) To be
published as part of the *Psychology, Religion, and Spirituality Series*,
Westport, CT: Praeger/Greenwood. (Harold J. Ellens, series editor).

Rogers, Diane. (2004, January/February). The Gospel Truth. *Stanford*,
Vol. 32, No. 1, pages 51–55.

Rossi, Ernest: (1986). *The Psychobiology of Mind-body Healing: New Concepts of Therapeutic Hypnosis*. New York: Norton.

Ruck, C. A. P. , J. Bigwood, B. D. Staples, R. G. Wasson, and J. Ott (1979).
Entheogens. *Journal of PsychedelicDrugs*. Vol. 11, Nos. 1–2, pages
145–146.

Ruck, Carl A. P., Blaise Staples, and Clark Heinrich (2001). *The Apples of
Apollo: Pagan and Christian Mysteries of the Eucharist*. Durham, NC:
Carolina Academic Press.

Ruck, Carl A. P. (2003, Jan. 20). Was There a Whiff of Cannabis About
Jesus? *The Sunday Times* [London]. Available online:
    http://www.thehempire.com/pm/comments/281_0_1_0_C/.

Rudgley, Richard (1993). *Essential Substances in Society: A Cultural History
of Intoxicants in Society*. New York: Kodansha International.

Saunders, Nicholas, Anja Saunders, and Michelle Pauli (2000). *In Search
of the Ultimate High: Spiritual Experience Through Psychoactives*. London: Trafalgar Square/Rider.

Schultes, Richard Evans: (1976). *Hallucinogenic Plants*. New York: Golden
Press, pages 25–26.

Schwartz, Jeffrey M. and Sharon Begley (2002). *The Brain and the Mind:
Neuroplasticity and the Power of Mental Force*. New York: HarperCollins
Publishers.

Shanon, Benny (2002). *The Antipodes of the Mind: Charting the Phenomenology of the Ayahuasca Experience.* Oxford University Press.

Shulgin, Alexander 'Sasha' and Ann Shulgin (1991). *PIHKAL: A Chemical Love Story.* Berkeley, CA Transform Press.

Shulgin, Alexander 'Sasha' and Ann Shulgin (1997). *TIKAL: The Continuation.* Berkeley, CA Transform Press.

Smith, Huston (2001). *Cleansing the Doors of Perception: The Religious Significance of Entheogenic Plants and Chemicals.* New York: Tarcher/Penguin Putnam.

Smyth, J., M. C. Ockenfels, L. Porter, C. Kirschbaum, D. H. Hellhammer, and A. A. Stone (1998). Stressors and mood measured on a momentary basis are associated with salivary cortisol secretion. *Psychoneuroendocrinology.* May; Vol. 23, No. 4, pages 353–370.

Stanford, Barbara (1972). *Myths and Modern Man.* New York: Washington Square Press.

Sternberg, Robert J. (1988). *The Triarchic Mind: A New Theory of Human Intelligence.* New York: Penguin.

Stolaroff, Myron (1994). *Thanatos to Eros: 35 Years of Psychedelic Exploration.* Berlin: Verlag für Wissenschaft.

Stolaroff, Myron (1999). Are Psychedelics Useful in the Practice of Buddhism? *Journal of Humanistic Psychology,* Vol. 39, No. 1, pages 60–80.

Stone, A. A., C. A. Macro, C. E. Cruise, D. A. Cox, and J. M. Neale (1996). Are stress-induced immunological changes mediated by mood? A closer look at how both desirable and undesirable daily events influence sIgA antibody. *International Journal of Behavioral Medicine,* Vol. 3, pages 1–13.

Stone, A. A., H. Valdimarsdottir, L. Jandorf, D. Cox, and J. M. Neale (1987). Evidence that secretory IgA antibody is associated with daily mood. *Journal of Personality and Social Psychology,* Vol. 25, No. 5, pages 988–993.

Stone, A. A., J. M. Neale, D. Cox, A. Napoli, H. Valdimarsdottir, and E. Kennedy-Moore (1994). Daily events are associated with a secretory immune response to an oral antigen in men. *Health Psychology,* Vol. 3, No. 5, pages 440–446.

Strassman, Rick (2001). *DMT: The Spirit Molecule: A Doctor's Revolutionary Research into the Biology of Near-Death and Mystical Experiences.* Rochester, VT: Park Street Press.

Tart, Charles: (1969). *Altered States of Consciousness: A Book of Readings.* Garden City, NY: Doubleday.

Tart, Charles (1975). *States of Consciousness.* New York: E. P. Dutton.

Tart, Charles (1991). Influences of Previous Psychedelic Drug Experiences on Students of Tibetan Buddhism: A Preliminary Exploration. *The Journal of Transpersonal Psychology,* Vol. 23, No. 2, pages 139–174.

Tendler, Stewart and May, David (1984). *The Brotherhood of Eternal Love.* Panther paperback edition.

The Economist (2005). Pharmacogenomics: The Agony and the Ecstasy. March 10.

Tupper, Kenneth W. (2002). Entheogens and Existential Intelligence: The Use of Plant Teachers as Cognitive Tools. *Canadian Journal of Education: Revue canadienne de l'education.* Vol. 27, No. 4, pages 499–516.

Tupper, Kenneth W. (2003). Entheogens & Education: Exploring the Potential of Psychoactives as Educational Tools. *Journal of Drug Education and Awareness,* Vol. 1, No. 2, pages 145–161.

Ullman, Montague, Stanley Krippner, and Alan Vaughan (2002). *Dream Telepathy: Nocturnal Extrasensory Perception.* Charlottesville, VA: Hampton Roads Publishing.

Valdimarsdottir, H. B and D. H. Bovbjerg (1997). Positive and negative mood: association with natural killer cell activity. *Psychology and Health,* Vol. 12, pages 319–327.

Valdimarsdottir, H. B. and A. A. Stone (1997). Psychosocial factors and secretory immunoglobulin A. *Critical Reviews in Oral Biology and Medicine,* Vol. 8, No. 4, pages 461–474.

Wallace, Bob. (1997). *Horizon: Psychedelic Science.* Program No. 60/LSF/A611A. BBC-TV, Headfirst Facilities, 0171-287-2011. Broadcast 13th January.

Walsh, Roger (1983). Psychedelics and Self-Actualization. Chapter 10 in Grinspoon & Bakalar 1983.

Walsh, Roger and Charles S. Grob (eds.) (2005). *Higher Wisdom: Eminent Elders Explore the Continuing Impact of Psychedelics,* Albany, NY: State University of New York Press.

Walsh, Roger and Vaughan, Frances (1993). *Paths Beyond Ego: The Transpersonal Vision.* Los Angeles, CA: Jeremy P. Tarcher/Perigee.

Warshow, Robert. (1964). *The Immediate Experience: Movies, Comics, Theatre and Other Aspects of Popular Culture.* New York: Doubleday/Anchor.

Wass, Lane (2000). *Imagine that! Awareness Through Imagery.* Rolling Hills, CA: Jalmar Press.

Watts, Alan (1963). The Individual as Man/World. *Psychedelic Review,* Vol. 1, No. 1, pages 55–65.

Weinstock, C. (1983). Psychosomatic elements in 18 consecutive cancer regressions positively not due to somatic therapy. *American Society of Psychosomatic Dentistry arid Medicine Journal,* Vol. 30, No. 4, pages 151–155.

Whybrow, Peter C. (2005). *American Mania: When More Is Not Enough.* New York: W. W. Norton.

Wilner, Harry (1977). *Epic Dreams and Heroic Ego.* Zurich: Spring Pub.

Wilson, Edward (1998). *Consilience: The Unity of Knowledge.* New York: Alfred A. Knopf

Winkelman, Michael (2000). *Shamanism: The Neural Ecology of Consciousness and Healing.* Westport, CT: Bergin & Garvey.

Wolfe, Tom. (1968). *The Electric Kool-Aid Acid Test*. New York: Farrar, Strauss and Giroux.

Wulff, David (1991). *Psychology of religion: Classic and contemporary views*. New York, NY: John Wiley and Sons. Page 639.

Index

179, 180, 181, 182, 183, 184, 192, 195, 196, 202, 203

experiences, ix, xii, xiii

experiment, 68, 81, 83, 119, 146, 153, 155, 184, 194

experimental philosophy, 81

experimental theology, 81, 168, 182, 194

explanation, 127

exploration of ideas wherever they lead, 157

explorers, 6, 103, 116, 136, 137, 154, 156, 180

expression of needs, 90

extending the human mind, 109

extroversion, 6

Eysenck, Hans, 177

Facilitation of Religious Experience, 76

fairy tales, 20, 22, 23, 24

faith, 95

false hope syndrome', xi

fana, xii

fasting, 70

fear, 7, 33

fear, xi

feelings, 1, 5, 6, 34, 35, 36, 37, 38, 39, 56, 57, 58, 59, 62, 68, 71, 78, 79, 81, 83, 84, 87, 88, 91, 93, 94, 95, 135, 137, 139, 141, 180, 181, 195, 196, 205

Fetzer Foundation, 59

Fight Club, 46

fighting spirit, 90

financial community, 203

Flashbacks, 87

flow, 141

fluency and flexibility of ideation, 122

Folger Shakespeare Library, 8

folk tales, 2, 20, 22

formal operational, x

Forte, Robert, 70

Foundations of Psychedelic Studies, 45, 47, 49, 66, 79, 103, 107

Freedman, Daniel X., 5

Freud, 32, 33, 40, 46, 116, 140, 179

frightening, 6, 7, 30, 121, 136, 181

From Molecules to Mystery, 194

fun and humor, sense of, 176

Future of the Body, 117

future, 1, 6, 7, 8, 10, 11, 14, 47, 55, 81, 87, 103, 105, 116, 121, 148, 152, 154, 156, 158, 159, 169, 174, 175, 177, 186, 192, 196, 197, 198, 202, 206, 208

future, x, xiii, xv

G. W. Pharmaceutical, 204

Gardner, Howard, 120, 121, 166

generalizations, 143, 148, 150

generalizations and theories, multistate standard for evaluating, 152

generalizations in psychology, the social sciences, and education, 143

genes, 198

genetic-based reactions, 107

genius, ix, x

geniuses, ix

Gloaming, Milton, 87

global crises, xiv 207

Glock, M. H., 85

Gnostic gospels, 93

God, 18, 59, 69, 70, 76, 94, 195 within, 181

Goldstein, Kurt, xii

Goleman, Daniel, xi, xv

Good Friday Experiment, 76

graduate, 20, 58, 91, 92, 158, 175, 185, 187, 189 education, x school, 3 students, 174

grandiosity, 3

Greece, 169

greed, 205

Greer, George, 57

Grinspoon, Lester, 57, 75, 96, 145

Grof, xii, 1, 20, 21, 22, 24, 26, 28, 29, 32, 33, 34, 36, 37, 40, 45, 46, 47, 49, 50, 102, 103, 107, 108, 139, 183, 192, 193, 204, 205

Grof's map of the human mind, diagram, 28

Gross, A., xv

group support, 89

group therapy, 90